ESSENTIALS OF INDUSTRIAL DERMATOLOGY

To 'H.J.W.' in recognition of his enthusiastic encouragement.

Essentials of Industrial Dermatology

EDITED BY

W.A.D. GRIFFITHS
MA, MD, FRCP

AND

D. S. WILKINSON
MD, FRCP

BLACKWELL SCIENTIFIC PUBLICATIONS

OXFORD LONDON EDINBURGH

BOSTON PALO ALTO MELBOURNE

Editorial offices:
Osney Mead, Oxford, OX2 0EL
8 John Street, London, WC1N 2ES
23 Ainslie Place, Edinburgh, EH3 6AJ
52 Beacon Street, Boston
Massachusetts 02108, USA
667 Lytton Avenue, Palo Alto
California 94301, USA
107 Barry Street, Carlton
Victoria 3053, Australia

First published 1985

Set by Setrite Ltd, Hong Kong
and printed and bound
in Great Britain by
Whitstable Litho Ltd, Whitstable, Kent

DISTRIBUTORS

USA
Blackwell Mosby Book Distributors
11830 Westline Industrial Drive
St Louis, Missouri 63141

Canada
Blackwell Mosby Book Distributors
120 Melford Drive, Scarborough
Ontario M1B 2X4

Australia
Blackwell Scientific Book
Distributors
31 Advantage Road, Highett
Victoria 3190

British Library
Cataloguing in Publication Data

Essentials of industrial dermatology.
1. Occupational dermatitis
I. Griffiths, W.A.D. II. Wilkinson, D.S.
616.5 RL241

ISBN 0-632-00924-1

Contents

Contributors

D. BURROWS MD FRCP, *Consultant Dermatologist, Royal Victoria Hospital, Belfast BT12 6BA*

R. D. H. BURSELL LLB MA DPhil, of Lincoln's Inn, Barrister, *Guildhall Chambers, Broad Street, Bristol BS1 2HG*

R. CHURCH MA MD FRCP, *Consultant Dermatologist, The Royal Hallamshire Hospital, Glossop Road, Sheffield S10 2JF*

J. A. COTTERILL MD BSc FRCP, *Consultant Dermatologist, The General Infirmary at Leeds, Great George Street, Leeds LS1 3EX*

E. CRONIN FRCP, *Consultant Dermatologist, St John's Hospital for Diseases of the Skin, Lisle Street, Leicester Square, London WC2H 7BJ, and Honorary Senior Lecturer, Institute of Dermatology, London*

W. A. D. GRIFFITHS MA MD FRCP, *Consultant Dermatologist, St John's Hospital for Diseases of the Skin, Lisle Street, Leicester Square, London WC2H 7BJ, and Honorary Senior Lecturer, Institute of Dermatology, London*

T. C. HINDSON, MA, MB, BChir, MRCP FRCPEd DTM&H, *Consultant Dermatologist, Royal Infirmary, New Durham Road, Sunderland SR2 7JE*

R. J. G. RYCROFT MA MB BChir MRCP DIH, *Consultant Dermatologist, St John's Hospital for Diseases of the Skin, Lisle Street, Leicester Square, London WC2H 7BJ, and Honorary Senior Lecturer, Institute of Dermatology, London*

D. S. WILKINSON MD FRCP, *Formerly Consultant Dermatologist, Wycombe General Hospital, High Wycombe, Buckinghamshire*

D. M. WILLIAMSON MD MBChB Hons MRCGP MFOM DIH, *Consultant Dermatologist, The General Infirmary, Pontefract, West Yorkshire WF8 1PL*

Preface

Industrial dermatology as a subject is less than a century old. The Industrial Revolution reached its zenith half a century earlier, and the need for knowledge and expertise in the field of dermatology related to industry became ever more keenly felt in our industrial areas, until the challenge was taken up by a general practitioner in Wigan who had a few dermatological sessions. Dr R. Prosser White published in 1915 the first monograph on the subject. Unfortunately, even today most doctors who have the responsibility of dealing with industrial dermatology problems, both factory medical officers and dermatologists, receive little or no formal training in the subject. This book is primarily intended to meet the needs of the factory medical officer with no specialized knowledge of dermatology. We hope that this volume will also provide those in formal dermatological training with a useful introduction to the subject.

All our contributors have been selected for their experience of working in industrial areas, and throughout we have encouraged a direct practical approach of setting some of the problems of industrial dermatology in the wider context of dermatology in a population of working age. We have deliberately not attempted to cover all aspects of this very specialized subject.

We wish to express our grateful thanks to our many colleagues who have generously given us time and advice in all stages of the preparation of this work.

Keypoints appear at the end of chapters, in italic type.

Chapter 1
Industrial Dermatitis — a National Problem

W. A. D. GRIFFITHS

Great Britain is one of the leading industrial nations. It is therefore surprising that of 240 British dermatologists only a small handful have taken a special interest in industrial dermatology. In 1915, Dr R. Prosser White, a general practitioner in Wigan, published a major treatise on the subject, *The Dermatergoses or Occupational Affections of the Skin*. His lead was followed by a few enthusiasts who took the first steps in establishing an industrial dermatology service in this country (Wilkinson 1980). In fact, Scandinavian dermatologists showed an even earlier interest in the subject than British ones. Recognition of the need for a greater intensity of effort in industrial dermatology is beginning to be accepted, partly from a greater awareness of the size of the problem and partly due to the economic implications resulting from sickness in industry. Governmental legislation and pressure from the trade union movement have also provided some impetus to the study of the skin in an industrial context. In a recent survey among dermatologists in training, many of them expressed the need for more instruction in industrial dermatology.

Dermatological disease occupies a very special place among those conditions responsible for time lost from employment. In many instances the problem is preventable, and in the remainder there is a better than average chance of improving the patient sufficiently to allow his quick return to work. The challenge of industrial dermatology can be appreciated by examining the size of the problem from figures which are available to us in the annual statistical returns of the Department of Health and Social Security (DHSS 1981). Whilst one has to accept that caution is required in interpreting the data, they do provide us with information which shows the overall patterns of disease and often reveals some surprises.

Table 1.1 gives an estimate for 1978 for the numbers at risk from industrial disease.

Table 1.1. Group estimates for the numbers at risk from industrial disease (1978)

Total work force	25 million
Pensioners	8.6 million
Non-working women and children	16.4 million

Prevalence of sickness

Spot checks of returned sickness certificates show that on any one day there are about *one million* people off sick. This figure refers only to certified sickness. Since in Britain the first 3 days of any spell of sickness are counted as waiting days and are not certifiable, the actual number of people off sick at any one time can be considered to be in excess of two million.

About 25% of the population at risk (i.e. the working population) make a sickness claim per year, two-thirds of them being for one period of sickness, but a fifth claiming two spells per year. In 1978 this amounted to 220 million working days lost to industry. This enormous figure acquires even greater significance when the economic implications are considered. There is the cost to industry of the loss in productive capacity, there is the cost to the taxpayer of very large sums in sickness benefit. Sickness benefit alone accounted for nearly £100 million in 1978. Unemployment and industrial disputes add an additional and increasing economic burden.

As many doctors are unaware of the categories of sick persons and the types of benefit which are currently payable, some notes on these topics are given.

The first three 'waiting days' are not certifiable and do not count for benefit. The following groups are excluded:

(a) the elderly;

(b) members of the Armed Forces;

(c) mariners while at sea;

(d) most non-industrial civil servants and Post Office employees (who do not normally claim sickness benefit until an illness has lasted 6 months);

(e) married women and certain widows who have chosen not to be insured for sickness/invalidity benefit.

Groups (b), (c) and (d) are not entitled to injury benefit. The *self-employed* make up another important excluded group as they are not insured for industrial injury.

Statutory Sick Pay

From 6 April 1983, most people who work for an employer and pay Class I National Insurance contributions will not get State Sickness Benefit for the early weeks of sickness. Instead they get 'Statutory Sick Pay' (SSP) from their employers. The first 3 days of an illness are counted as waiting days for which no benefit is payable. The upper rate payable in 1984 was £40.25 per week. After 8 weeks the payment normally stops and the sick person may be entitled to transfer to Sickness Benefit.

State Sickness Benefit

The current rate of State Sickness Benefit is £25.95 for a man under 60. This amount may be increased by £43.50 for a husband and wife, and other increases are available. By contrast, the unemployment benefit basic rate is £27.05.

Invalidity Benefit

This is made up of an invalidity pension of £32.60 plus a small supplementary invalidity allowance. It is paid in place of sickness benefit if the person continues to be incapable of work after 28 weeks, and continues up to the age of 65 for men or 60 for women.

Industrial Injury Benefit

This was abolished in April 1983 and was replaced by Statutory Sick Pay for the first 15 weeks. For certain prescribed industrial diseases, currently numbering 49, an industrial disablement benefit (see below) may be payable. That relating to dermatology is Prescribed Disease D5 (formerly PD 42), defined as 'non-infective dermatitis of external origin (including chronic ulceration of the skin but excluding dermatitis due to ionising particles or electro-magnetic radiations other than radiant heat)'.

Industrial Disablement Benefit

From 15 weeks after contracting an industrial prescribed disease, Industrial Disablement Benefit may be paid. The degree of impairment is normally assessed by a doctor experienced in industrial problems and is expressed as a percentage disablement. The rates payable range from £55.60 for 100% to £27.80 for 50% and £5.56 per week for 10% or less. If the disablement is 20% or less the benefit is generally paid as a lump sum.

Since this industrial disablement benefit is payable in addition to the ordinary invalidity benefit, the worker will be better off if his dermatosis is judged to be industrial. The doctor's certification of Prescribed Disease D5 should only be made after careful consideration.

Constant Attendance Allowance

This is an allowance for people who are so seriously handicapped that they need constant care and attention as a result of the effects of an industrial accident or disease.

Exceptionally Severe Disablement Allowance

This refers to an increase where the constant care and attention is liable to be permanent.

Unemployability Supplement

If, because of the results of an industrial accident or disease, a patient is likely to be permanently unable to work, he may be entitled to an increase in his Industrial Disablement Pension. It is currently £32.60 per week.

'Other employees may become restive and a panic situation may seriously disrupt the working capacity of the factory. Small factories without their own medical officers cause problems not easily identified since the individual workers report to different general practitioners who are usually not aware that other workers are similarly affected.'

Effect of age

Unlike most other specialities, the maximum impact of skin disease is on the younger age-group. This can be seen clearly in Fig. 1 which indicates that the maximum number of certified spells off

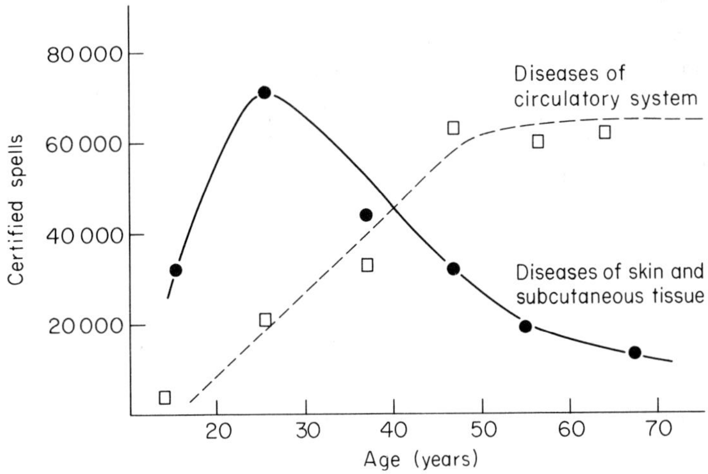

Fig. 1. Spells of certified sickness against age, 1977/8.

work for skin diseases occurs amongst 20- and 30-year-olds. For comparison, circulatory diseases are also shown to have a steadily increasing incidence with age. A most important factor emerges when the number of days actually lost is examined as opposed to the number of spells off work. For dermatological diseases the number of days lost is low and remains so with increasing age. By contrast, diseases of most other systems cause a considerable and

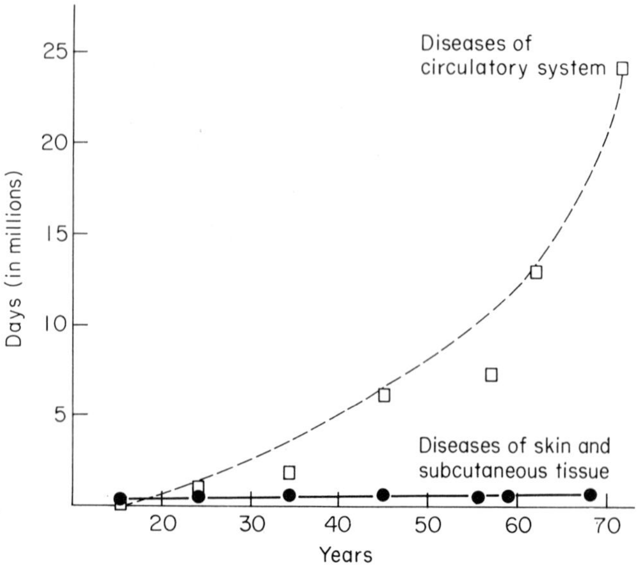

Fig. 2. Days of certified sickness against age, 1977/8.

steadily increasing loss of working days with increasing age (Fig. 2). It is clear from these two figures that it is possible by early diagnosis and treatment to improve the condition of patients with skin disease and return them back to work, in contrast to the degenerative disorders.

Regional variation

Industrialization varies in different parts of Britain but areas with economic and social problems tend to show a higher degree of morbidity not wholly accounted for by the level of industrialization and population densities. Two health service regions shared the position for the highest number of certifications for industrial dermatitis with almost double the national average. These were the North West and Yorkshire & Humberside regions.

Trends

Newhouse (1972) pointed out that the number of days lost from industrial dermatitis had fallen between 1953 and 1969 by 40% but

Table 1.2. Days of work lost from industrial dermatitis (D5), males only

1953/4	780,000
1971/2	400,000
1977/8	200,000

still exceeded the number due to all other prescribed diseases by the ratio of nearly 3:1. This trend has been continued but has levelled off at 25% of the 1953 level (Table 1.2). It is not clear whether the fall is due to more discerning diagnosis of industrial dermatitis or whether it is a genuine fall due to greater awareness of industrial hazards to the skin.

The present position is far from satisfactory, however, as *industrial dermatitis in 1977/8 accounted for 75% of days lost for all prescribed diseases.*

How may things be improved further?

The establishment of the International Contact Dermatitis Research Group (ICDRG) has helped to pinpoint new dermatological hazards in industry at an early stage before the problem has become widespread and has sometimes enabled a small change in technology to avoid the hazard completely. It has also focused attention on the industrial aspects of dermatological practice. Malten *et al.* (1971) reported on 4000 patients with eczema from five European centres participating in the ICDRG and found that industrial dermatitis accounted for 19.1% of all cases seen, excluding housewives' dermatitis. They emphasized that the figures were likely to underestimate the risk to certain groups such as the self-employed who tend to tolerate their dermatological problem until they are forced to stop work.

Several centres in Great Britain have established specific industrial dermatitis clinics. Wilkinson, Budden & Hambly (1980) have collected figures from their own experience over 10 years, and found that of the patients referred to them with possible industrial dermatitis the diagnosis was probably correct in 70%. The proportion of irritant to allergic contact dermatitis varied widely according to the industry. In engineering they found 60 irritant dermatitis cases to 21 allergic, and in hairdressing 12 irritant to five allergic. The proportion was reversed in other industries such as furniture manufacture with 36 irritants to 75 allergic, and in the rubber and plastics industry with nine irritants to 25 allergic. Fifty per cent of their patients gave one or more positive reactions when tested to the ICDRG Standard Battery of patch tests. Interpretation of the results can sometimes be very difficult (see Chapter 3).

Certain individuals seem particularly prone to develop skin problems in industry. Hannuksela (1980) reported on the susceptibility of atopic subjects. He suggested that atopic individuals coming into contact with foodstuffs may develop a variety of cutaneous reactions including contact urticaria with a typical weal and flare, but also a dermatitis resembling other types of contact dermatitis. The place of constitutional skin disease in industry is considered in Chapter 4.

Progress may be expected if current interest in industrial dermatology is maintained. The special needs are for more accurate identification of the risk factors, (a) in the external working environment and, equally as important, (b) in the susceptibilities of individual types of skin. Zschunke (1980) has stressed five principles for the better management of industrial dermatitis which we fully endorse. They are:

1 improvement in technology
2 improvement in personal protection
3 elimination and replacement of noxious materials
4 legislation
5 information and instruction

Information

Any social security office is able to provide the following useful pamphlets for more detailed information:

NI 196 Social Security Benefit Rates
NI 16 SSP and Sickness Benefit
NI 16A Invalidity Benefit
NI 2 Industrial Injuries: Prescribed Industrial Diseases
NI 6 Industrial Injuries: Disablement Benefit and Increases
NI 10 Industrial Injuries: Industrial Death Benefits

References

Department of Health and Social Security (1981) *Social Security Statistics, 1979*. Her Majesty's Stationery Office, London.

Hannuksela M. (1980) Atopic contact dermatitis. *Contact Dermatitis*, **6**, 18–19.

Malten K.E. *et al*. (1971) Occupational dermatitis in five European dermatological departments. *Berufsdermatosen*, **19**, 1–14.

Newhouse M. L. (1972) Sickness absence due to industrial dermatitis. *Transactions of the St John's Hospital Dermatological Society*, **58**, 48–50.

White R. P. (1915) *Occupational Affections of the Skin*, 1st edn. H. K. Lewis, London.

Wilkinson D. S. (1980) The challenge of industrial dermatitis. *Clinical and Experimental Dermatology*, **5**, 327–38.

Wilkinson D. S., Budden M. G. & Hambly E. N. (1980) A 10-year review of an industrial dermatitis clinic. *Contact Dermatitis*, **6**, 11–17.

Zsunchke E. (1980) Management of industrial dermatitis. *Contact Dermatitis*, **6**, 18–19.

- *There is no room in industrial dermatology for hurried consultation, skimped history-taking, or guesswork.*
- *The diagnosis of industrial dermatitis may carry implications far beyond those of the individual patient.*

Chapter 2
Industrial Dermatitis Today and its Prevention

D. BURROWS

Prevention of industrial dermatitis is important for the factory doctor for the following reasons.

1 It is by far the commonest industrial disease. The incidence varies in different countries from 20 to 80%. In the United States, contact dermatitis accounts for 58% of all industrial diseases.

2 Contact dermatitis can produce severe disability and work impairment. An appreciable percentage of people who develop contact dermatitis in industry will never be completely and permanently cured.

3 The social status and future work prospects of a worker are affected if he develops a long-standing dermatitis. It has been shown in West Germany that over 60% of those who develop industrial dermatitis suffer financial loss.

4 The development of dermatitis in a factory can be a cause of friction between management and industry. Many doctors may be unaware that workers have a deep-rooted suspicion of dermatitis due to anxiety about unemployment and ability to work in the future. The unknown is feared. The introduction of a new process causing skin reactions produces great anxiety among workers. Furthermore, unions are taking an increasing interest in dermatitis, its prevention and, in particular, compensation of their members. This has both a good and bad effect. Management may be unaware and unconcerned about skin problems in a particular process, and it may only be after pressure from the union or mounting costs of litigation that any steps are taken to solve the problem. It can also lead to an earlier involvement of the medical profession in a situation in which dermatitis is occurring in a factory and this is only to be welcomed. There is, however, the problem of increasing litigation. Though this may have a beneficial effect in forcing a firm for financial reasons to improve a work process where dermatitis is occurring frequently, it may also lead to employers becoming

reluctant to employ workers with a history of dermatitis. A worker may have a flare-up of his dermatitis and in turn claim against the firm. The present industrial injuries awards system does not adequately cover loss of wages or allow for pain and suffering, hence the incentive to claim under common law (see Chapter 1). Compensation awarded by the courts under common law is based on the adversarial system which does nothing to help industrial relations.

5 Because of increasing litigation, employers' liability insurance is becoming more expensive. In some areas of the country where there are industries with a relatively high incidence of dermatitis, the premium to cover dermatitis claims can add 10–20% to wages expenses. Anything, therefore, which prevents development of dermatitis in industry or reduces its incidence, will not only improve the general health and comfort of the workers, reduce costs and make industry more efficient, but may indeed improve industrial relations.

Interest was stimulated in the problems of contact dermatitis by the formation of the International Contact Dermatitis Research Group (ICDRG) in 1967 which brought together interested dermatologists from seven European countries, now increased to nine. It arose from the Scandinavian Committee for Standardization of Routine Patch Testing, which had spent 5 years meticulously examining the variables encountered in the patch test procedure and establishing preferred sites and techniques. Since its inception, the ICDRG has held meetings in 12 different countries at 6-monthly intervals. On five occasions the ICDRG has held international symposia during which participants from many countries have presented short papers on the subject of contact dermatitis.

The work of the ICDRG began with an epidemiological study of 4825 patients, the first large-scale computerized study of its kind carried out in this field. Its results formed the basis of six joint publications between 1969 and 1972. The study of individual allergens, potential or established, has formed an important part of the work of the group, drawing, as the members can, on joint series of 1000–2000 patients every 6 months. It includes a reappraisal of techniques, assessment of the reason for changes in annual figures of sensitizing chemicals, and the recognition and appraisal of new allergens, whether occupational or domestic. The Standard European Battery (SEB) is continually being re-examined and improved (see Appendix 3). The group has recently concerned itself with the very difficult problem of irritancy.

Among many publications deriving from the ICDRG, there must be mentioned the valuable small textbooks on patch testing by Drs S. Fregert and H. J. Bandmann, and *Contact Dermatitis*, the journal of environmental and occupational dermatitis, edited by C. D. Calnan, which is now in its 11th year. This is indispensable for any dermatologist or occupational health physician working in the field of contact or occupational dermatology (see Appendix 1).

But perhaps the most lasting achievement of the ICDRG has been the stimulus it has provided to the formation of the national groups devoted to this important aspect of dermatology:

North American Contact Dermatitis Group (NACDC)
Belgian Tri-Contact Dermatitis Group
Groupe d'Etudes et de Recherches en Dermato-Allergologie (GERDA)
Groupe Espanol Investigacion Dermatitis Contacto
Contact Dermatitis Research Group (CDRG) in Comecin
MID-Japan Contact Dermatitis Research Group
Allergen Research Group of Japan
British Contact Dermatitis Research Group

In the industrial field Scandinavian countries have been particularly prominent, and the first university department of industrial dermatology was founded in 1960, in the University of Lund, with Dr S. Fregert as head. In Sweden there are currently nine dermatologists in different departments engaged full-time in industrial dermatology. In Britain there are two — Drs Richard Rycroft and Ian White at St John's Hospital, London. In 1980 a new British Contact Dermatitis Research Group was founded to co-ordinate and promote research into contact and industrial dermatitis in Britain.

Causes of dermatitis in industry

With the development of new products and the decline of older industries, the causes of dermatitis and the industries in which it most commonly occurs change from time to time. The incidence of dermatitis in industry differs between males and females and Appendix 2, by Dr Fregert, gives a list of occupations in order of importance in which dermatitis occurs and the common allergens and irritants in these industries which produce dermatitis. It can be seen that there is a different pattern of cause and industry for males and females. This is due entirely to the different occupation pattern of women and not due to any physical differences between the sexes (for British figures, see Chapter 1). Almost 80% of cases of dermatitis in industry are caused by primary irritants.

Prevention of dermatitis

There are four areas which may contribute to a reduction in the incidence of dermatitis:

1 Factory management
2 Worker responsibility
3 Engineering skills
4 Medical suspension

1 Factory management

Warnings

If a worker is in contact with a substance which has the potential to irritate or sensitize the skin, it is essential that he should be warned about this and given advice about how to prevent it happening. The duty of the factory is accepted generally, medically and legally and a factory may be considered negligent if personnel are not warned about substances they are handling which are known to be dangerous to the skin. These warnings can take the following forms.

1 *Notices* which are posted in the factory, very often beside the washing facilities. Cautionary placards which are available from Her Majesty's Stationery Office (HMSO), and which are relevant to the skin are as follows:

Chrome — effects on the skin (ref. SHW 395)
Dermatitis — workers in contact with flour, dough or sugar (ref. SHW 355)
Synthetic resins (ref. SHW 366)
All industries (ref. SHW 367)
Lemon and orange peeling, effects on the skin (ref. SHW 396)

The Royal Society for Prevention of Accidents (RoSPA)

produces a durable instruction plaque which can be nailed to the wall beside the wash basins. The following Health and Safety Executive Advisory Publications are helpful (HMSO):
Dermatitis — effects on the Skin of Mineral Oil (ref. SHW 295)
Industrial Dermatitis and the Worker (ref. SHW 2064)
2 If the worker is in contact with substances which have a high potential for injury to the skin, such as epoxy resin, cement, oils, acids and alkalis, then the warning may need to be more specific and personal, in the form of a verbal warning to the operator which may take the form of a pre-induction lecture, or a hand-out given specifically to the workman indicating company policy about handling the materials, the use of washing facilities, protective clothing and emollient creams. It is not sufficient to make protective rules and inform the staff; one must see they are complied with.

Labelling

Industrial data sheets should be readily available for inspection and all chemicals used on the site listed. All packages of chemicals should be labelled with their contents and advice about use.

Washing facilities

It is generally accepted that for all work where there is a risk of dermatitis there should be at least one wash-hand basin or 2 feet of washing space for every 10 persons. Where materials handled are strong irritants or sensitizers there should be at least one wash-hand basin or its equivalent for every five persons employed.

The following Health and Safety at Work booklets are very helpful:
Cloakroom Accommodation and Washing Facilities, No. 5
Industrial Dermatitis; Precautionary Measures, No. 18

Drying is equally important. Roller towels are not satisfactory, for in spite of good intentions, they may not be changed often enough and remain constantly wet and dirty. There are three acceptable alternatives:
1 disposable paper towels;
2 pulldown-type roller towel;

3 hot air drying — if workers are using a substance which has a tendency to degrease the skin, a hot air drier may aggravate this problem and should only be used in conjunction with an emollient cream to apply after use.

The choice of a hand cleanser is important and will depend on the type of work in the factory. Soap and water will be suitable for most purposes. Cleansers containing paraffin oil and volatile organic solvents should be avoided unless there is some very special indication for their provision. It is widespread practice for workers to clean their hands with the solvents used in the process or for cleaning machines. These will almost certainly be strong degreasers and irritants of the skin, and this practice must be actively discouraged, along with the common use of bleach in a dye house to remove colours from stains on the hands. Occasionally, special purpose solvent or abrasive cleansers may be needed, but they should only be provided for specific purposes and then used intermittently.

Barrier and emollient creams

It is now generally accepted by the medical and legal professions that barrier creams have no protective function on the skin, and recent evidence would suggest that they may indeed facilitate penetration of the skin by irritants. Occasionally, dermatitis has even developed to the barrier cream itself (see Chapter 10). They may, however, have some use in allowing easier cleaning of the skin where there is excessive soiling. A far more important provision is for emollient cream to be applied after washing or at the end of the day, and this is especially important where operatives are handling substances which are likely to degrease the skin.

Protective clothing

The need for protective clothing and the type supplied depends on the following factors:

1 the irritant and sensitizing potential of the substances with which the operatives are in contact;

2 the frequency with which they are in contact;

3 contact with other substances which may predispose to irritation and sensitization, for instance, constant wetness;
4 whether or not there is airborne contact.

Gloves. The constant wearing of impervious gloves can itself cause maceration and increase the vulnerability of the skin to dermatitis. It may be more harmful to wear impervious gloves in domestic work where water and detergents get inside the gloves than not to wear gloves at all. Some chemicals have been shown to penetrate rubber gloves (e.g. methyl chloride [used in paint stripper], methyl methacrylate, phenolformaldehyde resin, nickel sulphate, 20% neomycin in soft paraffin, epoxy resin, and nickel) and polyvinyl chloride gloves (methyl chloride, epoxy resin, and turpentine peroxide). Therefore, any benefit from wearing gloves must be balanced against the possibility of potential irritation, as the use of gloves can produce a false sense of security. Many other substances, particularly when dissolved in solvents, can penetrate rubber gloves in half an hour and the penetration can continue when the gloves are not in use. When this occurs with maceration under an occluded glove, a high index of irritation results. The use of protective gloves is discussed further in Chapter 9.

Where there is danger of oil scattering over the body, particularly on the thighs, where oil folliculitis may be a problem, or on the scrotum, an impervious apron should be worn. If there is airborne dust, as with fibreglass, boiler suits should be supplied and it is most important that these should be laundered regularly and not together with household clothes.

2 Worker responsibility

The ultimate responsibility for prevention of dermatitis must lie with the worker himself. Good housekeeping and general cleanliness at the work bench and area are vital in this. Gloves should not be left around to become contaminated, and should be removed in such a way that the offending substances do not get on the inside of the glove. If the factory does not launder the boiler suits, it is essential that the operative himself should regularly launder his protective clothing before it becomes too soiled. This would be particularly important in circumstances where there is contact with oil and fibreglass so that the oil does not soak through to the trousers which he will wear on the way home.

3 Engineering skills

Minimized handling

This is probably the area where reduction in the incidence of dermatitis can be most achieved in the future and already automation is producing an improvement in dermatitis statistics. A good example of this is the change in the way cement is mixed mechanically — centrally rather than by hand on site. This is probably responsible for the considerable reduction in cement dermatitis in the past few years. Necessity is a great improviser, and in some cases automation has not been installed until dermatitis has occurred, and the resulting improvement may lead not only to reduction in dermatitis but increased productivity. There should be no hesitation in encouraging increased automation for a process where dermatitis is a high risk, such as handling of epoxy resins, chemicals, solvents and degreasing agents.

Use of Non-dermatitis-producing products where possible

A good example of this is replacement of chromate by other anti-rust agents. Unfortunately, chromates are still widely used in industry for this purpose, a use which should be strongly discouraged. Trivalent chromate plating should be used instead of the usual hexavalent chromate plating. This has the double advantage of producing less dermatitis and being a much better environmental agent because it is less toxic in the environment. Recently, it has been shown that the addition of small amounts of ferrous sulphate to cement will reduce hexavalent to trivalent chromium, which is less sensitizing. This could be added at manufacturing level and is being considered in some countries, or it may be used where operatives are at most risk, when mixing and working with wet cement. It could also be added to the water. Diesel oil is best avoided in mould oil for cement casting. When advising against the use of certain products, one must ensure that more dangerous ones are not substituted. For instance, because of some dermatologists' reports of parabens sensitivity, many manufacturers of local applications have changed to other preservatives which may have an even greater sensitization potential.

Environment

In situations where an allergen or an irritant occurs in the environment, good ventilation is essential. There are three main areas where this is particularly important.

1 *Plating.* It is important here to have ventilation suction in close proximity to the area of plating to remove noxious cyanide fumes and also chromate and nickel in the atmosphere which could sensitize.

2 *Fibreglass.* In many fibreglass operations, particularly where there is sawing of fibreglass treated with epoxy resin, there is a very dense fine dust of fibreglass in the atmosphere which gets into clothes and produces intense itching. Most people become hardened to this but some develop a chronic dermatitis.

3 *Epoxy resin systems* give rise to fumes. The resin itself, the catalyst, the additives and epoxy diluents may sensitize. During curing, some systems release halogen gases which are primary irritants. The problems are intensified if the process requires heat to hasten curing or to alter the viscosity. Ventilation in the area in which the resins are mixed should be of the highest efficiency and close to the operative area. The large resin producers offer a service to industry in re-designing plant to overcome hazards of exposure.

It should be emphasized that a very large range of epoxy systems is currently available. Low molecular weight epoxy resins are now the main sensitizers.

4 Medical suspension

Pre-employment examination

Those workers with a type of skin which would predispose to dermatitis should be discouraged from taking up occupations where they are likely to come into prolonged contact with irritants. Persons with dry skin or eczema are more liable to irritation and contact dermatitis. It is important, therefore, that workers who are exposed to irritants should have a pre-employment medical examination. The application form should include questions about previous skin trouble including dermatitis. At the pre-employment examination, the prospective employee should be specifically asked about any previous history of eczema or 'dry skin' and the examination should include positive examination of these conditions. A tendency to seborrhoeic eczema will be aggravated by hot or damp conditions. If this is a risk, a special search should be made for seborrhoeic eczema and this will have to include examination of the body folds, such as the groin, perianal area and axillae as well as the scalp and ears. Heavy soiling of the skin with oil can produce oil folliculitis due to blocking of the hair follicles and sebaceous glands by oil. People with a tendency to acne are more liable to develop this condition and it is not advisable to employ a person with severe acne in an occupation where there is going to be heavy oil contact. Pre-employment patch testing should not be performed as a routine. It can lead to sensitization and will not identify those who will become sensitized. If there is any special doubt, this can usually be resolved by history taking or resort to the patient's doctor or a dermatologist's opinion. If doubt still persists that the prospective employee may be allergic to some substance he is going to handle, e.g. nickel or epoxy resin, then a patch test may be helpful but it should be carried out by a dermatologist, unless the factory doctor has some special training or expertise.

Good medical facilities

There are four aspects to medical care of the skin in industry.

1 *The factory medical officer* is the person of prime importance. It is important that the medical officer, even though he only has a part-time contact with the factory, should know intimately all the processes in the factory and should have an awareness of where the risks for dermatitis lie. A good factory medical officer will need to have a slightly more than average knowledge about skin diseases in order to make an accurate diagnosis at an early stage. The medical department should encourage all workers with skin problems to report to the department at an early stage. The longer contact

dermatitis continues, the more chance it has of becoming chronic and persisting even when the patient is removed from the source. It can be very difficult to distinguish an irritant contact dermatitis from allergic contact eczema after a period of time. Many cases of contact dermatitis in industry are precipitated by an injury in the following way: (a) the injury may become infected and develop an infective dermatitis and go on to a contact dermatitis; (b) the barrier of the skin may be coping very well with the irritants with which it is in contact and keeping them from penetrating the skin but the injury overcomes this barrier and allows the irritants to penetrate and trigger off dermatitis; (c) many cases of contact dermatitis develop through inappropriate treatment in medical first aid. It is important not to use substances for dressings which are liable to sensitize the skin, e.g. antihistamine creams, acriflavine, merthiolates, etc. For first degree burns it is unnecessary to apply anything more than a bland preparation, such as calamine cream or E45 cream, and for deeper burns or abrasions, a bland tulle, such as a Jelonet or Melolin dressing should suffice.

2 The *GP* should be informed at an early stage of any skin problems in order that treatment may be continued at home. It may be that there is some other previous skin condition or family problem, about which the factory medical officer is unaware.

3 If there is any doubt about the diagnosis of a skin condition the patient should be referred to a *dermatologist*. When a skin condition has gone on for some months it may be difficult even for an expert to distinguish between constitutional eczema and contact dermatitis. It is essential to make an exact diagnosis at an early stage. Most dermatologists would be very willing to help and indeed there is usually at least one in each area who has a special expertise in industrial skin problems. Most dermatologists would welcome and benefit by an invitation to visit the factory where the skin problem has occurred.

4 The *Employment Medical Advisory Service* was established in 1973 and incorporated into the Health and Safety at Work Act in 1974. Under this Act, the Health and Safety Commission and the Health and Safety Executive were set up. The former consists of a chairman and nine members drawn from both sides of industry and local authorities. Its function is one of general responsibility for health in industry and it may initiate special investigations into

problem areas. The Executive has three members and under its direction the Health and Safety Inspectorate and the Employment Medical Advisory Service. The Employment Medical Advisory Service has two main functions:

(a) advising people with health problems about the type of work which suits them or which they should avoid on health grounds;

(b) helping to prevent ill health caused by work.

Dermatology has a special relationship with the Employment Medical Advisory Service (EMAS) in that there is a joint health service and part-time EMAS dermatology post at St John's Hospital, Lisle Street, London. Where there are special problems which may be particularly baffling, for instance, an outbreak of skin disease in a factory where no obvious cause exists, it may be helpful to obtain the special expertise of EMAS.

- *Skin reactions following the introduction of a new process can cause great anxiety in the workers.*
- *Employers' liability insurance may add 10–20% to overheads.*
- *The International Contact Dermatitis Research Group has been founded to collate experience and stimulate research.*
- *Management has a responsibility to advise the workers of the hazards to which they are exposed. Posting of warning notices is not sufficient.*
- *Industrial solvents should not be used to clean the hands.*
- *Barrier creams are inefficient as barriers.*
- *Simple changes in handling routines are often effective against high-risk procedures.*

Chapter 3
Investigation of Industrial Dermatitis

C. HINDSON

Large firms usually regard their medical officer as part of the management team, and as such he should have access to all confidential information on manufacturing processes with particular regard to adhesives, resins, woods, oils and other chemicals in use. Dermatitic hazards of such chemicals are readily gleaned from a comprehensive text (see Appendix 2) and will not be covered in detail here. The industrial medical officer is, therefore, more likely to encounter the sporadic case rather than the epidemic. In the event of the latter situation, it is important to remember that while trade names of substances in use may remain the same, suppliers sometimes alter or add to a product without changing these.

The factory visit

This is a must. If you are part of management no problem exists, but if visiting on a 'hostile' basis, great care and tact are necessary.

Decide what is important to see and see it, without diversion, while also inspecting what management or the workforce may also think relevant.

Cautious deliberate deviation from the proposed inspection route can often yield useful clues.

The author has devised the mnemonic VATICAM for anyone new to the subject:

Ventilation
Air extraction
Tidiness
Illumination
Cautionary notices and procedures
Ablution facilities
Motivation and attitude of work force

Assessment of these seven factors will give a good background to the works before assessing the specific problem.

Ventilation

This must be seen to be adequate and working. It may be important to take a humidity and temperature reading as some non-specific skin complaints have been associated with low humidity.

Air extraction

This is separate from ventilation, and individual processes where fumes are generated — such as hot epoxy resin operations — need individual extractors. Volatile agents need to be handled in fume cupboards with protection for the hands.

Tidiness

This gives an immediate indication of the level of general discipline in the work force. Particular attention should be paid to spillage of liquids, contamination of workers, and storage of tools and substances not in use.

Illumination

Adequate illumination is vital as a general safety measure, but remember there have been reports of light-induced dermatitis from fluorescent strip lights.

Cautionary notices and procedures

General notices warning about dermatitis, and specific notices where known dermatitic substances are in use, must be prominently displayed.

Employers are required by law to ensure that whatever protective clothing is necessary is readily available and adequate for the purpose. They are also required to ensure that workers know what the hazards are and why they have to wear protective clothing.

Ablution facilities

The standard of cleanliness, supply of cleansing agents, and appropriate notices on their use are indications of the care taken by management for its workers.

Check that primary irritants such as paraffin and dieṣel oil are not in use as skin cleansers.

Over-dependence on barrier creams should be discouraged (see Chapter 10).

Motivation

General conversation with the employees usually reveals the extent of this. Multiple trivial complaints may indicate low morale or sometimes an impending attempt to increase 'danger' allowances in the next round of wage talks.

Conversely, good morale on highly rewarded tasks may lead workers to disobey safety regulations or hide dermatitis, or both.

The industrial case history

It is important to be familiar with the process from which the dermatitis is alleged to have arisen. This will enable you to ask relevant questions and help prevent involvement in a long discussion with the patient in his own technical jargon.

The following questions should always be asked.

Previous history

1 Is there a history of atopic disease (asthma, eczema, hayfever)? The answer 'Yes' here suggests that the skin disease may be constitutional, at least in part.
2 Has he had dermatitis in a previous job? If 'Yes', what was the nature of the job? It may be that he first contacted the allergen in that job.

Present job

1 How long has he been doing it?
2 How long was it until dermatitis developed? Remember allergy can occur after many years in the same job.
3 Have any new substances been introduced?
4 Are any other workers affected? Who works with him and is without skin trouble?
5 Who, if anyone, has treated his complaint? Sometimes there is

additional contact eczema from medicaments such as antihistamines purchased at the local chemist.

6 How much pay has been lost? This is a very important question and the answer may give the reason for the complaint. Where no work has been lost, there may be a motive for a disability pension or the union may be using the case to alter working conditions or pay structure.

Hobbies and part-time jobs

Enquiry must be made into these. The author recently investigated a case of hand dermatitis in a machine operator who turned out to be a keen gardener allergic to primula plants.

The examination

The whole of the skin must be examined and not just the area of complaint. This will often reveal the basic nature of the disease. Patches of psoriasis elsewhere may suggest that the hand dermatitis in that case was endogenous with only minimal exacerbation attributable to industrial oils.

Industrial rashes are commonly eczematous although there are several notable exceptions. They tend to occur on areas of maximum exposure. Where the hands and feet are affected the dorsal surfaces show more involvement than palmoplantar areas where the skin is thicker.

Where the distribution of the rash is unusual, remember the possibility of defects in protective clothing. Rashes on face and neck suggest contact with a vapour or aerosol.

Microscopic examination of skin scrapings for fungus is essential, particularly with chronic scaly rashes of hands and feet. Indeed, ringworm is reasonably held as a disability that merits compensation in some hot, wet occupations, such as coal mining.

Dermatitis of finger-webs and sides of adjacent fingers often occurs as a primary irritant reaction to metal swarf in cutting oils.

Patch testing for allergy

Closed patch testing has become an accepted procedure to detect the cause of acquired allergic contact dermatitis.

Success in patch testing is analogous to prowess in sport; only those who play the game regularly excel at it. The uninitiated should take lessons or leave it to the regular players. The International Contact Dermatitis Research Group have developed a Standard European Battery of 20 of the commonest allergens which are listed in Appendix 3.

To produce uniformity most dermatologists obtain their test materials from one source (Associated Hospital Supply, PO Box 4, Pershore, Worcestershire WR10 14), though a similar standardized range has recently become available (Dome-Hollister-Stier, Strawberry Hill, Newbury, Berkshire RG13 1JA).

Technique

The usual patch tests are a series of filter paper discs attached to aluminium foil strip (Al Test, Imeco, Asda Chemicals, Watford WD1 7QR). An alternative system uses concave aluminium discs mounted on acrylic adhesive paper (Finn Chambers, Associated Hospital Supply, PO Box 4, Pershore, Worcestershire WR10 14J). In this, a small slither of the reagent is applied to the paper disc. Strips of reagents are then applied in vertical rows to the patient's back on either side of the spine and affixed with paper tape (Dermilite, Johnson & Johnson, or Micropore MMM).

The skin next to each patch is then marked for recognition with a felt-tipped pen (Staedler Lumocolor 315 is satisfactory), or alternatives. Some clinics then apply a close fitting vest to ensure the patches are not rubbed off (Essiban, size 30 cm, E. Sallis Ltd, Nottingham). The vest and strips are removed at 48 hours, and the results are recorded ½–1 hour later. This delay is to allow tape reactions to subside.

Although a 48-hour reading is often considered adequate to detect most sensitizers, this is not reliable and some substances, notably neomycin and even nickel and bichromate, may only give positive reactions at 72 or 96 hours. If it is not possible to carry out a second reading at 96 hours a single reading at 72 hours is preferable to one at 48 hours. The patches must, however, be removed by the patient at 48 hours and the sites of application must therefore be marked.

'False negative' tests at 2 days only are the cause of medico-legal disputes, but 'false positive' reactions are even more likely to be misinterpreted and become the cause of unnecessary restrictions on the worker.

A false irritant positive reaction is usually confined to the area of the test and, if severe, may show a flaccid bulla or superficial necrosis. It seldom shows the typical spreading vesicular and oedematous reaction of the true allergic response, but some reaction between these extremes may be distinguished with difficulty, even by experts in patch test interpretation (see Table 3.1 for grading system).

Table 3.1. Reading patch tests

−	(Negative) No reaction
±	Doubtful positive
+	Positive
++	Strong reaction (erythema with oedema and vesiculation)
+++	As for ++ but spreading beyond the test site

Finally, always keep meticulous notes of the nature and concentration of the substances tested, its diluent (if any) and an exact description of any positive reaction observed.

Unexpected positive and negative results are both commonly seen. Some of the causes are listed below.

False positive reactions

1 Concentration of test substance too high or it is a primary irritant.

2 The patch was contaminated with another substance prior to application.

3 Several unrelated substances give positive results. This is known as the 'angry back syndrome'. The substances should be retested separately a few weeks later. Patients should not, in any case, be tested when their dermatitis is in an acute phase.

4 The patient has irritated the patch himself — artefact may occur when compensation is a factor.

False negative reactions

1 The wrong substance was tested.
2 The concentration was too low.
3 The test site was recently treated with topical steroids. (Patients taking more than 20–30 mg daily of prednisolone will not give reliable patch test results.)
4 Insufficient allergen was released. This usually happens when pieces of clothing are tested.
5 The patch was not properly applied or came loose.
6 Reagent became inactive through age.
7 Slow reactivity (e.g. neomycin may be negative at 48 hours, but positive at 96 hours).
8 Reagent suspended in inappropriate vehicle.
9 Accidental misorientation of test strips.

Any test procedure carried out on human subjects depends upon interpretation. Differences between individuals can be reduced by careful attention to approved techniques but can never be eliminated. This is especially true of reactions to irritants. Correctly carried out, patch testing affords a reasonably reliable guide to allergic sensitization, though reactions resulting from past immunological 'scars' must be distinguished from those likely to be of current relevance. For instance, some 12% of all adult women in this country are likely to have acquired nickel sensitivity from ear-rings, jewellery or jeans buttons.

In general, therefore, patch testing is best carried out in a clinic devoted to this and by those experienced in applying, reading and interpreting the tests. An increasing number of dermatological units in district general hospitals have, or are acquiring, such facilities. In large cities, there is usually one centre which has a well-equipped industrial or contact dermatitis unit (e.g. St John's Hospital for Diseases of the Skin, London). At such units, the expertise is enormous and appropriate dilutions of individual ingredients (and other cross-reacting allergens) are likely to be available or easily obtained. In this way, a precise indication of a particular sensitivity may be obtained. Moreover, such testing may be linked with enquiries — or even visits — to a factory in which several workers may have been affected, if the management or industrial medical officer so desires.

'Aimed' patch testing (e.g. the application of one or more substances to which a worker may appear to be 'allergic' is, however, often carried out at the factory or in the doctor's surgery. For the reasons stated clearly above, this practice is best avoided; but if it is attempted, great care must be taken to observe the following guidelines.

Patch testing with unknown substances

It is tempting to test with some liquid or dust which the patient believes to be the cause of his dermatitis. This is a hazardous procedure.

Never perform a closed patch test on an unknown industrial agent. Find out, first, if it is a strong acid or alkali; if so, do not test at all. If it is of a solvent nature, or a moderately weak potential irritant, which has been handled by the worker, you can easily carry out a simple 'dab' test or — for weaker substances — a repeat usage test twice a day for 3–5 days. The substances should be applied to an area no bigger than a 10 pence piece, just below the elbow flexure. The site should be inspected each day. At the most, this is only likely to give information about possible irritancy.

Many substances are primary irritants and one should never contemplate patch testing with diesel oil, petrol, detergents, or lubricating oils, because severe bullous reactions may occur. Cutting and cooling oils produce irritant dermatitis and where an allergic reaction occurs it is often to an additive such as an antimicrobial and not the oil itself (Chapter 7).

If these tests are negative, a closed patch test may be carried out at, first, 1/10 the usage dilution. But a positive result may still only indicate a (weaker) irritant effect on this particular worker. Nevertheless, it may be a helpful indication of an irritant that has penetrated a worker's gloves and remained on the skin for some hours.

Remember that the conditions of a closed patch test are much more rigorous than open contact with a substance for 5 or 6 hours per day. As a general rule, no *unknown* substance should be tested at a greater concentration than 10%. One notable exception is sawdust which is applied neat ('as is' is the patch test phrase for neat).

To determine allergic sensitization, it is necessary to apply the suspected allergen or component of a mixture at a recognized dilution (see below) that does not cause an irritant reaction. This dilution may be extremely low, e.g. 0.1–0.2% isopropyl paraphenylene diamine, or quite high (to ensure penetration), e.g. 12% parabens mix or 30% wool alcohols ointment.

Application of strong sensitizers in inappropriate strengths may cause active sensitization, which is often revealed by a 'late' reaction at the patch test site 7–21 days after application. This risk must be avoided in any worker likely to be in contact with this allergen in the future.

Always read the test yourself. Do not leave this to a nurse. The patient should be instructed to take the tests off ½–1 hour before reading, to avoid confusion with the 'stripping' reaction and to allow pressure effects to subside. If more than one test is applied, a skin marker will be needed. Thirty per cent dihydroxyacetone in acetone, a 'caramelling' agent, is widely used. Gentian violet, brilliant green or similar paints remain in place for 2 days, though there is a very slight risk of sensitization to the last. Do not use red or green ball-point pen. Blue or black are allowable but may have to be coated with 'Nobecutane' or 'New Skin' to avoid being washed off in bathing.

Notes on some of the reagents in the European Patch Test Battery (see Appendix 3)

Metals

Nickel sulphate 5% in pet (yellow soft paraffin)

This is the commonest sensitizer in women, and initial sensitivity is usually acquired domestically from jewellery, wrist watches, bra clips, studs in jeans, zips, coins in pockets, and ear-rings. In men, nickel allergy was usually occupational in origin but recently more is being seen in young men from jean studs and ear-piercing.

Nickel sensitivity becomes a problem for nurses and hospital cleaners who have to handle nickel-containing objects in circumstances where the skin may also be damaged from chemical irritants and detergents.

Patients with nickel sensitivity are prone to develop chronic hand eczema.

Nickel can be detected in metal by the nickel spot test. The test object is moistened with ammonia water and two drops of 1% alcoholic dimethylglyoxime are added. A pink colour develops in the presence of nickel in a concentration down to 1 in 100,000.

Potassium dichromate 0.5% in pet

This is the commonest sensitizer in men and among the top 10 for women. Its occurrence is widespread in industry. Chromate sensitivity is commonly acquired where other factors are also operating to damage the skin. Thus cement damages skin due to its alkalinity and abrasiveness and chromate sensitivity is acquired although the chromate content of cement may only be 20 parts per million.

Once acquired, chromate eczema tends to run a chronic course even though the patient may leave the job in which it developed. This may be due to the universality of chromate in the domestic environment. Chromate sensitivity may be acquired from cement, foundry sand, grinding processes, paint, paint primers, dyes, dust from metal sanding, rust preventives, corrosion inhibitors in cooling systems, textile dyeing, match heads, electric arc welding, chrome plating, chrome tanning of leather, and finished leather. A more exhaustive list should be consulted if necessary (see Further Reading List).

Cobalt chloride 1% in pet

Cobalt is not a common industrial allergen but has been reported from use in printing inks, in paint pigments for pottery, china and plastics and in papermaking.

Cobalt frequently cross-reacts with nickel and gives positive patch tests in patients who are allergic to nickel.

The rubber chemicals

Paraphenylene diamine mix (PPD)

Although these chemicals are rubber accelerators, one is also a black dye used in rubber, leather, and also as a hair dye. Patients allergic to sulphonamides may also react to it. It is particularly valuable in picking up occupational sensitivity to phenylisopropyl-p-phenylenediamine in black rubber of tyres, hoses, etc.

Thiuram mix, mercapto mix, carbamate mix

These three test reagents are each made up of four derivatives of each class of accelerator and constitute the commonest sensitizers in rubber.

In addition, the mercapto group (MBT) may be found as preservatives in canvas to prevent mildew, as sprays for fungus in gardening and agriculture, and as a preservative in antifreeze and cooling systems.

Antibiotics/antiseptics

Neomycin 20% in pet

This is usually acquired from prolonged topical applications.

Quinoline mix 0.01% in pet

Quinoline used as a topical antimicrobial in several medicaments. Sensitization may depend on the extent of local use.

Bases/preservatives

Wool alcohols 30% in pet

Allergy generally develops from long-continued application of ointments (as opposed to creams), particularly in leg ulcer patients.

Ethylene diamine 1% in pet

This substance is widely used in industry but it is not a frequent cause of dermatitis. It is used as a corrosion inhibitor in antifreeze solutions, in polyamide resin adhesives, in electroplating solutions.

It has caused dermatitis when added to cooling oils. The commonest reported causes of dermatitis from this chemical are from its use as a stabilizer in a popular medicament cream.

Parabens 15% mixture in pet

A group of preservatives added to many cosmetic and medicament creams.

Balsam of Peru 25% in pet

Occurs in soaps, chocolate, orange peel, various scents and perfumes, shaving creams and toothpastes. Its constituents may be relevant to perfumes in soaps and cosmetics.

Others

Turpentine peroxides 0.3% in olive oil (now omitted from the routine list)

These active agents are obtained by steam distillation of various species of pine trees and are known as gum spirits of turpentine. They contain various terpenes which are built up from isoprene units

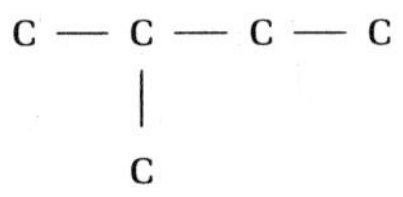

to form monocyclic terpenes such as lemonene, pinene and carene and their isomers. These are difficult substances to separate chemically. Natural turpentine is not now widely used and has been largely replaced by aromatic petroleum biproducts such as white spirit (mineral turpentine, turps substitute).

Oil of turpentine, however, also contains substances used in perfumery — geraniol, citronellol, menthol and terpinols.

Formaldehyde 2% in water

Allergy to formaldehyde is less common than the above-listed allergens but when detected on patch testing its origin may be difficult to trace.

It is used 'as is' in laboratories, but allergy may arise from substances which break down to release formaldehyde such as biocides added to cutting oils, formaldehyde polymer resins used in drip dry, non-crease, and retext clothing, phenolformaldehyde resin adhesives, urea formaldehyde-based glues, nitrogenous agricultural fertilizers, offset printing processes.

Colophony 20% in pet

Colophony is the residue left after distillation of pine gum rosin. Allergy to it until recently has usually been from application of surgical adhesive tapes in which it was used for its adhesive properties. Newer tapes (Dermilite, Johnson & Johnson) have acrylic-based adhesives so that colophony allergy from this source will decline. Colophony also occurs in insulating tapes, glues, varnishes, sealants and surface coatings, glue size, soldering flux, shoe and furniture polish, some cutting oils, medicaments, linoleum, chewing gum, and some clear soaps.

Epoxy resins

These are widely used in industry as adhesives, insulators, hard-wearing paints, in liquid form in the manufacture of some PVC handbags and in backing of some PVC adhesive tapes. They consist of two components — the resin and the hardener or curing agent which brings about polymerization of the resin monomer.

Allergy usually develops to the resin, possibly due to its epoxide grouping

```
    O
   / \
— C — C —
```

Allergy to the hardener is much less common. Allergy to the cured resin does not occur but reactions may occur to impurities of uncured monomer still present.

An important clue in the history is that the patient will usually know that two substances (the resin and hardener) have to be mixed together shortly before the process takes place. This puts the odds very firmly on an epoxy origin and patch testing with the ICDRG reagent will usually produce positive results. It is important to ensure that the right molecular weight epoxy is used for testing.

Caine mix

A mixture of procaine, cinchocaine, amethocaine, cyclomethocaine and benzocaine. The high sensitizing potential of topical local anaesthetics, particularly from over-the-counter sales, makes this group an important component of the Standard Battery.

p-Tertiary butyl phenol formaldehyde resin 1% pet

This is widely used in neoprene adhesives bonding the soles of shoes. It is also used as a sealant in the car industry and in various glues.

Perfume ('fragrance') mix

A mixture of the eight most common sensitizers in perfume. The best and simplest indicator of perfume sensitivity that is available. Musk ambrette in male cosmetics has recently been recognized as an important cause of allergy.

- *Patch tests incorrectly performed or interpreted may raise further medico-legal complications.*

Chapter 4
Constitutional Skin Disease in Industry

J. A. COTTERILL

Introduction

It is important that the industrial medical officer recognizes and has some knowledge of the more common skin diseases, for two main reasons. First, the presence of certain skin disorders will preclude work in a number of occupations, and secondly, a large proportion of patients with what they imagine may be industrial dermatitis turn out to have constitutional skin disease. For instance, in a recent survey, 29% of patients referred to an industrial dermatitis clinic were found to have skin diseases which were considered non-occupational in origin (Wilkinson, Budden & Hambly 1980).

There are five common skin diseases that may pose problems in industry in Great Britain. These are acne vulgaris, psoriasis, gravitational eczema and ulcers, atopic eczema, and tinea pedis.

In this section we shall consider the grevalence and principles of diagnosis of these disorders, the selection of the work force, and the types of work that may be hazardous to those affected.

Acne vulgaris

Prevalence

Almost all normal adolescents have some degree of acne, the peak age of incidence being 14 years in females and 16 years in males. Fortunately, only about 10% of adolescents develop severe acne, and when this occurs, in both sexes, the affected individuals often continue to have problems well into the third decade. Between 5 and 10% of females still continue to develop some acne lesions until the menopause.

Diagnosis

Fortunately, acne is easy to diagnose. The clinical picture is polymorphic. The face is almost always involved. The skin is excessively greasy and is characterized by the presence of blackheads, whiteheads, papules and pustules, and in severer cases cysts, nodules and scarring. In individuals with severe acne, both the back and upper chest are commonly involved.

Work force selection and types of work hazardous for employees with acne

It has long been known that acne is exacerbated by a hot, humid environment. Thus, it is no coincidence that Shakespeare's only description of a character afflicted by acne was of a kitchen worker (Cotterill 1972). It is now thought that sweating may indirectly reduce sebum excretion. This effect may be due to an increase in hydration of epidermal and pilo-sebaceous keratin in particular, leading to a reduction in the size of pilo-sebaceous ducts and an increase in sebum outflow resistance. Increased hydration of keratin may also play an important part in the flare or premenstrual acne (Cunliffe & Cotterill 1975). From a historical point of view it is also interesting to note that tropical acne was a major cause of invalidism in the American armed forces in the Pacific theatre during the Second World War. The armed forces are thus reluctant to take recruits with extensive acne because these personnel may have to serve in a hot, humid environment and tropical acne then becomes a risk. Similarly, tropical acne may be provoked in the sort of working conditions found in a hot engine room in a merchant ship in the Persian Gulf. In females, hairdressing and kitchen work are also occupations prone to this complication and should be avoided if possible. Firm evidence that acne subjects are more prone to oil acne is lacking.

Psoriasis

Prevalence

There are no accurate figures on the incidence of psoriasis in Great

Britain, but it seems to be agreed that the prevalence in North-West European adults lies between 1.5 and 2% of the population (Baker & Wilkinson 1979). However, there are some racial variations and psoriasis is unusual in African negroes and in the Japanese. There are two peak ages of onset for psoriasis, one in childhood and one around middle-age. It is generally agreed that patients with a young age of onset and a strong family history of psoriasis carry a worse prognosis than those patients without these prognostic features.

Diagnosis

Psoriasis is one of the dermatological disorders that every medical practitioner is usually able to diagnose without difficulty. The patient with the common plaque form of psoriasis has red plaques distributed particularly over the extensor aspects of the body involving the elbows, knees and scalp. The plaques are well-demarcated and are usually scaly. The discoid lesions may coalesce in time into extensive plaques. Another common clinical variant of psoriasis is guttate psoriasis which is seen most often in children following a streptococcal sore throat, but occasionally also in adults following tonsillitis and also following episodes of severe emotional stress. In this variant the individual lesions are raindrop-like and usually 2–5 mm in diameter. This clinical type of psoriasis often has a good prognosis, especially in children.

Less well-recognized clinical features of psoriasis include persistent hyperkeratotic changes on the palms and the distal pustular type of psoriasis involving hands and feet. Nail dystrophy may also be seen, producing many nail abnormalities including pitting, onycholysis, yellow discoloration of the nail plate and even splinter haemorrhages. Patients with nail dystrophy tend to have a higher incidence of arthropathy. Reliable figures are not available for the incidence of arthritis in psoriasis, but most are agreed that about 15% of psoriatics may develop this complication.

Work force selection and types of work hazardous to employees with psoriasis

Most patients with psoriasis are able to lead a relatively normal life and to follow almost any occupation they may turn their mind to.

Fortunately, psoriasis very rarely affects the face and many individuals with the condition learn to disguise their skin with appropriate clothing. Thus women often wear trousers during the day and some patients even carry with them small portable vacuum cleaners so that they may remove any tell-tale scales that they may leave in their environment.

Psoriasis tends to be worse in humid and also in cold climatic conditions and both these environments should be avoided. On the other hand, sunshine and a dry sub-tropical climate improves most patients. The Koebner (isomorphic) phenomenon is important in an industrial setting and is quite common in patients with psoriasis. It occurs when an apparently clinically normal area of skin is traumatized, for instance by an abrasion or by a burn, with psoriasis developing at the injured site. This phenomenon may also be seen following primary irritant dermatitis of the hands, e.g. induced by soluble cutting oils or solvents.

Employment of the psoriatic in the health services, including contact with patients, is also open to some debate. Unfortunately, psoriatic skin in a hospital environment is very liable to be colonized by pathogenic organisms and particularly by pathogenic strains of staphylococci. The nurse, surgeon or anaesthetist with extensive psoriasis may cause outbreaks of hospital cross-infection. The writer considers it prudent to discourage people with extensive psoriasis or with a history of severe psoriasis from following those occupations which involve close contact with patients; others may consider such a policy unduly harsh. A flexible approach to the problem would seem the best advice.

Gravitational ulcers and eczema

Prevalence

Gravitational ulcers and eczema develop in legs affected by venous insufficiency. Capillary pressure rises because of valvular incompetence and these progressive changes may lead to the post-thrombotic syndrome. It must be stressed that varicose veins on their own do not necessarily produce dermatological pathology. The post-thrombotic syndrome is seen eventually in most patients following a deep venous thrombosis, and one survey showed that

45% of patients developed this syndrome within 5 years of a deep venous thrombosis and 91% after 10 years. The ankle perforators seem to be particularly troublesome, possibly because the capillaries around the ankle are subjected to a higher pressure than the capillaries at other sites in the leg. Either gravitational eczema or frank ulceration often finally develops in this area.

These pathological changes may be precipitated by several factors, but a new job involving much standing is a common cause, particularly in those who have had a venous thrombosis.

Diagnosis

The diagnosis of a gravitational ulcer is usually straightforward. Classicially the ulcer begins around the medical malleolus, perhaps with other physical signs such as varicosities, oedema, hyperpigmentation, or areas of 'white atrophy' where previous ulcers have healed. Ulcers occurring on other sites in the leg usually have a different pathogenesis. Arteriosclerotic or hypertensive ulcers tend to occur on the lateral aspect of the lower leg. Neoplastic ulcers can occur at any site, but squamous carcinomas are one of the rare late complications of long-standing leg ulcers.

Gravitational eczema

Gravitational eczema presents few difficulties in diagnosis. The patient usually has a red excoriated eruption, sometimes weeping, often scaly and maximal around the medical malleolus. Gravitational ulcers are commonly associated with gravitational eczema or medicament contact and eczema may spread to all body areas. If the skin is not completely examined, the correct diagnosis may be missed.

Work force selection and types of work hazardous to employees with gravitational ulcers or eczema

Any occupation involving prolonged standing is contraindicated in patients with gravitational eczema or ulcers. Some common examples of jobs involving prolonged standing are shop assistant, barman and barmaid, tailor, and many occupations in industry such as engineering work on lathes. An occupation that may involve trauma to the affected leg should be avoided, as gravitational ulcers often follow comparatively minor trauma to the medial malleolus of the post-thrombotic leg.

Atopic eczema

Prevalence

The term 'atopy' was introduced by Coca & Cooke in 1923 to define a group of patients suffering from eczema, asthma and hay fever. There is often a strong family history of these disorders. High titres of IgE (reagin) antibodies may be found in those severely affected by atopic eczema, but the precise part played by immunoglobulin in the pathogenesis of the eczema remains unclear.

The incidence of atopy in Great Britain is not known but various estimates have placed the figure between 2 and 20%. A recent survey in Northern Europe found an incidence of atopy of about 15% in the parents of newborn infants, and of 14.3% in the parents of 7-year-olds and about 15% in the 7-year-olds themselves. Of this 15%, about 8% had atopic eczema. The chances of an individual developing overt clinical symptoms are increased if one or both parents are atopic. Where both parents were atopic, over 40% of children were found eventually to develop atopic symptoms.

Most atopic individuals tend to improve with age, and by the time they reach employable age, will have lost most of the symptoms and signs of eczema, apart from some xeroderma. In a smaller group of patients however, atopic eczema may develop for the first time in the late teens, in middle or even old age.

It is important to remember that it is quite common for the predominant symptoms to change; as the eczema becomes less of a problem either asthma or hay fever may come to dominate the clinical picture, causing further (but different) problems with regard to employment.

Diagnosis

Diagnosis is usually straightforward in a typical case of atopic eczema, but the clinical features vary in severity with time. In teenagers and adults the most characteristic sites affected are the antecubital and popliteal fossae, the flexor aspects of the wrists, ankles and neck. Lichenification due to prolonged rubbing and scratching is also a feature. During exacerbations the skin may weep and become much more itchy. Some adults, particularly males, develop a light-sensitive eruption which is most marked on light-exposed areas such as the face and dorsal aspects of the hands.

Work force selection and types of work hazardous to employees with atopic eczema

It is now generally accepted that the constituted atopic is more susceptible than others to the development of primary irritant changes in the skin (e.g. Wilkinson 1980). An irritant may be defined as a substance which will produce inflammatory change in the majority of the population if applied in both sufficient concentration and for a sufficient length of time. Whilst there have been claims that the use of primary irritant substances like soap led to no significant changes in eczematous skin, it is known that normal skin at distant sites in patients with hand eczema is more susceptible to irritants than normal skin. Thus, the presence of eczema, and even recently healed eczema, tends to predispose a person to the effect of primary irritants.

It is also known that primary irritants cause occupation dermatitis more commonly than sensitizers. Wilkinson (1980) has found that this proportion varies with the industry, primary irritant dermatitis being common in engineering but less common in the furniture, electronic and rubber industries. Some patients may develop both primary irritant and then subsequently true allergic contact dermatitis; the irritated and damaged skin allows penetration of potential allergens. Sensitivity to rubber following the use of rubber gloves worn to protect the skin after an episode of primary irritant dermatitis is a common example; perfume sensitivity to scented head creams is another.

Thus subjects with atopic eczema and subjects with a past history of recent eczema and possibly even those with a history of atopic eczema as a child and a strong family history of eczema should avoid exposing the skin to potential primary irritants as much as possible. Repeated physical trauma should also be avoided.

The atopic should also avoid environmental factors which may induce itching, such as an increase in ambient temperature, extremes of relative humidity or a dusty atmosphere.

Occupations which present special risks include work involving exposure to coolant oil in the engineering industry, work involving exposure to mineral or diesel oil — for instance, employment as a fitter or car mechanic should be avoided and so should contact with paraffin, trichloroethylene and any other lipid solvents. It is important that the atopic does not work in extremes of humidity, high temperature, or excessively low temperature environments. It should also be remembered that protective clothing may also cause problems by increasing both local skin temperature and humidity.

Smallpox vaccination should not be undertaken in atopic subjects unless it is vitally necessary and then only under cover of gammaglobulin, but other inoculations are permissible. Atopic nurses and doctors are much more susceptible to the vaccinia virus than non-atopics. The same applies to the herpes virus, but the only occupation where this seems to be a problem is wrestling (herpes gladiatorum).

Atopic skin may be easily colonized by pathogenic organisms in a hospital setting and subjects with extensive eczema should be discouraged from choosing a career in either nursing or medicine. It may be possible by careful and frequent medical attention to get an atopic patient successfully through his or her training period.

Tinea pedis

The sharing of shower facilities and the necessity for wearing protective and therefore occlusive footwear make tinea pedis a common problem in industrial practice. In some occupations, such as mining and diving, the risk is especially great. Many workers accept tinea pedis and its associated malodour as normal and perhaps even as 'manly'. Since a wide range of effective topical antifungal agents is now available, the emphasis should be on prevention by encouraging improved personal hygiene, a high standard of public hygiene in common washing areas and occasional medical examinations.

Conclusion

Acne vulgaris, psoriasis, gravitational eczema, atopic eczema and tinea pedis are the commonest skin conditions encountered in the employable and employed population. Each of these disorders may pose special problems for the individual concerned and also for his employer. As long as care is taken over job selection, most individuals with even severe skin problems can be gainfully employed.

References

Baker H. & Wilkinson D. S. (1979) *Textbook of Dermatology*, 3rd edn (eds A. Rook, D. S. Wilkinson and F. J. G. Ebling), p. 1315. Blackwell Scientific Publications, Oxford.

Coca A.F. & Cook R. A. (1923) The classification and phenomena of hypersensitiveness. *Journal of Immunology*, **8**, 163–182.

Cotterill J. A. (1972) Shakespeare on the skin. *British Journal of Dermatology*, **86**, 533.

Cunliffe W. J. & Cotterill J. A. (1975) *The Acnes — Clinical Features, Pathogenesis and Treatment*. Saunders, London.

Wilkinson D. S. (1980) The challenge of industrial dermatitis. *Clinical & Experimental Dermatology*, **5**, 327–38.

Wilkinson D. S., Budden M. G. & Hambly E. N. (1980) A 10-year review of an industrial dermatitis clinic. *Contact Dermatitis*, **6**, 11–17.

- *Constitutional skin disease affects industrial workers and the general population with equal frequency.*
- *Hyperkeratotic psoriasis of the palms is often unrecognized.*
- *Complete exclusion of atopics from a workforce is both unfair and unnecessary,* but *care is needed in their job assignment.*

Chapter 5
Some Causes of Error in the Diagnosis of Occupational Dermatoses

D. S. WILKINSON

Constitutional diseases of the skin in relation to industry have been considered in the previous chapter. We believe it will be helpful to explore this relationship further by describing the experience and conclusions resulting from studying a large number of patients seen in an industrial skin clinic.

Over a 10-year period, 678 patients were referred to a special 'industrial' clinic attached to the department of dermatology in a district hospital in South-East England (Wilkinson, Budden & Hambly 1980). The area was one of relatively light industry but dominated by a traditional emphasis on furniture and paper manufacture. It was therefore only necessary to hold the clinic on one session a fortnight, but it served the purpose of being able to see and investigate all cases suspected of being of occupational origin without delay and to centralize information and records. The standard of general practice was high, but no less than 193 of the 678 patients were considered to have diseases that were not occupational in origin.

Dermatologists are certainly not exempt from error in this field. We frequently make mistakes — otherwise few cases would come to be disputed in Court — but they are chiefly in certain 'grey' areas such as the relative importance to be attached to constitutional or to occupational factors in patients with atopic dermatitis, or in the difficult situation in which a patch of discoid eczema follows some little time after an alleged splash of a chemical.

Table 5.1 shows the diagnoses that were made in the patients who were not thought to have occupational dermatoses. Let us consider some of the less important groups first.

Seborrhoeic dermatitis

Though the 'classical' patterns are easily recognized, seborrhoeic

Table 5.1. Diagnoses made in 193 patients referred to an industrial dermatitis clinic but not accepted as being occupational in origin

Eczema, all types	93	Seborrhoeic dermatitis	12
discoid	32	Psoriasis	9
vesicular, hand	20	Lichen planus	5
atopic	17	Urticaria, prurigo	14
leg/foot and spreading	9	Infection, infestation	5
other patterns	15	Fungal	4
Contact dermatitis,		Miscellaneous	31
non-occupational	20		

Reproduced from *Contact Dermatitis* (1980) **6**, 11–17, by courtesy of the editor.

dermatitis in the adult can merge into or be confused with atopic dermatitis or psoriasis. Occasionally occupational irritants, particularly dusts, can mimic some of the presentations of the disease, even causing some itching of the scalp. While investigating cases of sensitization to *Khaya* (West African mahogany), we observed a pattern of indeterminate erythema of the face or ears accompanied by a sensation of burning, which occurred in workers only in proximity to the dust but who were patch test-negative. At times, the symptoms suggested a mild seborrhoeic dermatitis, but the symptoms always faded very soon after leaving the factory.

The features of 'classical' seborrhoeic dermatitis are:

1 scaling, itching and perhaps crusting of scalp;
2 similar, though milder, scaling of eyebrows;
3 itching and scaling of the edge of the external auditory meati;
4 post-auricular erythema (close to fold);
5 spread to the sides of the nose;
6 a patch of fixed scaly erythema of the centre of the chest of men.

If any of these are present, the patient should be examined for intertriginous lesions in the axillae and groins, or follicular or scaly lesions elsewhere in the covered area. Marked eyelid swelling is not a feature of uncomplicated seborrhoeic dermatitis and points to an allergic contact dermatitis.

Seborrhoeic dermatitis is not an uncommon condition. The cause of the inflammatory stage is unknown. Susceptible or mildly affected individuals working in hot, humid or dusty conditions may occasionally be justified in believing that the condition would not have developed overtly had they not been engaged in such work. The history is important; the patient may forget episodes when the disease became active under quite different conditions. On balance, 'constitutional' factors, whatever they may be, are probably more important than environmental ones.

Psoriasis

It may at first seem surprising that this usually well-recognizable disease could be mistaken for an occupational dermatitis. But there are four circumstances in which it may. First, psoriasis may affect the hands exclusively, though this is rare, and tell-tale confirmatory spots are often seen on the elbows, knees or scalp on close examination. The knuckles are often involved and some finger-nails may show characteristic pitting. In other cases the psoriasis presents as a patchy hyperkeratosis of the palms or as a more diffuse psoriatic erythema. Secondly, this same change may occur as a result of the development of psoriasis on an area of pre-existing dermatitis, in a genetically predisposed person. This may pose difficult medico-legal problems if the patient pursues a claim for industrial benefit or compensation. At law, a person cannot be penalized for being a constitutionally determined psoriatic, any more than he can for having an 'eggshell skull' which splits when he is struck. The onus must, however, be on him and his doctor to show that the psoriasis would not have developed had he not been engaged on the particular work in question.

The third circumstance concerns the onset of psoriasis *de novo* on an area subject to industrial irritants or injuries. It is accepted that psoriasis may develop at the site of an injury as a 'Koebner phenomenon', e.g. at the site of a cut or an operation wound. In the case of an industrial irritant, it must be shown that both epidermis and dermis are injured and that the interval between the irritant exposure and the onset is reasonable. An interval of up to about 45 days may be allowable, but not longer; 10–30 days is more reasonable.

The fourth circumstance is the most contentious: the onset of an initial attack of psoriasis, usually generalized in type, following the assumed 'stress' of an injury, or of stress and anxiety arising from a particular occupation. The evidence that 'stress' can precipitate an initial attack of psoriasis is poor; that for the exacerbation of pre-existing psoriasis is more acceptable but must be subject to a stringent consideration of all the factors concerned. The disease is unpredictable in its behaviour and 'stress' is only too easily evoked in retrospect.

In the nine cases rejected in this series, there was considered to be insufficient evidence to associate the patient's psoriasis with his occupational exposure.

Lichen planus

This disease is normally so characteristic in its distribution that it would be difficult to confuse it with an occupational dermatitis. But, like psoriasis, it can occasionally arise as a 'Koebner' reaction at sites of injury.

A particular lichen planus-like eruption develops on the wrists of those handling photographic colour developers (CD2 [2-amino-5-diethylamineltoluene monohydrochloride]). Patch tests to 1% of the agent are positive but care must be taken to remove any chemical remaining after the test to avoid active sensitization (Fisher 1973). A similar lichenoid eruption has been recorded from contact with an anti-oxidant used in rubber tyres and by black stocking dye, but these are rare and exceptional. Lichen planus is almost always a non-occupational disease. Involvement of the oral mucosa should always be looked for.

Urticaria, prurigo

It is surprising that 14 patients with these conditions should have been referred to an industrial clinic. Acute urticaria is usually caused by food intolerance, drugs or injections containing foreign protein. Chronic urticaria is much more complex and the causes are almost always internal. There is a common belief among patients that it may result from detergents, sheets and other exogenous contacts but this is generally fallacious.

There are, however, two forms of chronic urticaria that may occasionally have an occupational context. The first concerns the physical urticarias — those due to sun and heat, cold and pressure. A careful history will elucidate most of these, but one is deceptive

— delayed pressure urticaria. This occurs at the site of pressure after some hours, usually about 7, differing in this respect from the other types of physical urticaria. We have seen it as a long unrecognized effect of carrying bags of cement on a shoulder in an otherwise healthy labourer. The second type is contact urticaria. This is often recognized by the patient but has undoubtedly been missed by dermatologists in the past. The diagnosis is made on the history of a burning redness and swelling of an area in contact with the responsible agent and which is reproducible by a '20 minute' occluded patch test. Some of the more common causes are listed in Table 5.2. Contact urticaria is prevalent in those handling shellfish, some vegetables and salads etc., and has caused some Danish open-sandwich makers to change their job. Atopic subjects are particularly vulnerable to this hazard.

The term 'prurigo' in Table 5.1 encompasses a group of conditions characterized by multiple excoriations or highly itchy

Table 5.2. Some occupational agents reported as causing contact urticaria

Non-immunological	Immunological (probable)
Alcohols	Acrylic monomer
Benzoic acid	Alcohols
Cinnamic acid and aldehyde	Alphate polyamides
Cobald chloride	Ammonia
Formaldehyde	Benzoic acid
Sodium benzoate	Diethyltoluamide
	Monoamylamine
	Nickel
	Platinum salts
	Plastic additives
	Polyethylene glycol

Uncertain
Ammonium persulphate

In addition, numerous foods and some plants, animals and textiles may elicit contact urticaria. These are important in certain special occupations, e.g. catering and food preparation, horticulture.

This is an incomplete list, abstracted from
Adams R. M. (1983) *Occupational Skin Disease*, pp. 60–61. Grune and Stratton, New York.

papules, usually involving the 'cape' area of the upper trunk and the extensor aspects of the proximal limbs. Most can be classified as neurotic excoriations, chiefly seen in depressed, middle-aged women. There is seldom any discernable relation with occupation, though mite infestation (more widespread and less regular) must be considered in cheese or straw handlers.

Infection, infestation

Table 5.1 shows that these were few in number. Occasionally scabies slips by and is presented as an 'occupational disease', perhaps because of the insistence of the patients on itching of the hands. The characteristic interdigital papules and excoriations and the burrows (when not scratched) should suggest the diagnosis and a full examination may reveal the characteristic penile papules in the male subjects. Prolonged infection may be accompanied (or followed by a non-specific eczema.)

Infections may, of course, be occupational in origin, e.g. anthrax or erysipeloid. But most infections of the skin presenting in this country are banal and not associated with work. There are, of course, a few specific exceptions, e.g. among hospital and mortuary workers.

Fungal infections

Primary involvement of the feet or groins would be uncommon sites for industrial dermatitis. But very specious explanations are often given to account for such eruptions. Splashing of chemicals or oils on to shoes may be acceptable but a vesicular eruption of the sole of one foot (especially) is much more likely to be fungal. Two of the four cases referred had a unilateral scaly eruption of one palm that was due to *Trichophyton rubrum* infection.

Other causes of contact dermatitis

Cases with undoubted contact dermatitis which was eventually not regarded as occupational in origin accounted for 10% of the erroneous diagnoses. This was in no way a reflection on the referring doctor; he was to be praised for recognizing the condition as an allergic contact dermatitis. But the decision as to whether the allergen is occupational or environmental may be a difficult one. What about nickel sensitivity, for instance? About 11% of all adult women are nickel-sensitive (D. S. Wilkinson, unpublished data, 1982). Most commonly this arises in adolescents from jeans buttons, wrist-watches, ear-rings or jewellery, or clothing clips. But this may be forgotten when a recurrence is associated with the handling of nickel-plated objects at work, especially in hot and humid conditions. There is some support for the view that secretaries, cashiers or hospital workers may be more at risk of developing such a sensitivity from handling objects at their 'work': but the evidence must be secure in view of the wide exposure of women to nickel in everyday life — similarly, colophony sensitivity may be of past relevance, relating to plaster sensitivity. Allergy to perfumes is also common in women and often missed if patch tests are not carried out. Medicament sensitivity is a common cause in both sexes and accounted for a quarter of all cases in this group. A man who blamed splashed oil for the rash on his legs was found to be sensitive to his trouser dye.

Patch tests are essential to the elucidation of this problem but must be carried out expertly and preferably in a unit that has considerable experience in this field (see Chapter 3).

The eczemas

Nearly half the cases which were thought to be of occupational origin were endogenous. It was this group that gave both us and the referring practitioner the greatest trouble and it is obvious that there is bound to be some difference of opinion about the role of exogenous irritants in all cases of eczema, whether these are occupational or environmental in nature. Bjornberg (1968) showed that once one area of skin became eczematous, others areas had a reduced resistance to irritants. Thus, an engineer in his mid-40s developed an irritant dermatitis of his hands, without change of work or oil, only after he had developed a patch of discoid eczema on his leg; which was to blame, the work or the discoid eczema? Leg or foot eczemas with secondary dissemination were seen in nine of the 93 patients.

Discoid eczema presents in two forms. In the first, which

particularly affects older men (and often those of managerial class or who are retired), a single patch of itchy, psoriasiform or perhaps exudative eczema appears on one leg. After an interval of from 10 days to several months, other patches appear in a symmetrical fashion, particularly involving the extensor aspects of the limbs. But aberrant forms or modes of onset or distribution are not uncommon. Though the essential cause is unknown, a dry skin or a low-humidity environment is often present (e.g. car heaters, blow heaters at home or in offices). Very rarely, the initial patch may follow contact with an industrial chemical irritant or sensitizer. The second form occurs equally in both sexes and affects young workers and the elderly worker whose skin is drying and who may be exposed to solvents or climatic chapping after work. Here, the discoid patches usually start on, and may be confined to, the dorsa of the hand. These we accepted as 'occupational' if an appropriate contact, e.g. over-washing by hairdresser apprentices or the use of solvents, was apparent. It is not yet clear whether atopic subjects are preferentially affected. In our material, this was the most common source of difficulty in referral: it is, perhaps, a form of eczema that is not well understood by non-dermatologists.

Hand eczema always causes difficulty. Since the hands are so important to a manual worker, time must be allowed at the first visit for a full history and a careful examination. The findings — especially the distribution of the eruption — should be carefully noted. Whereas eczematous patterns involving the backs of the fingers and hands or the pulps of the fingers are usually exogenous (but not necessarily occupational), palmar patterns are usually considered to be endogenous because of the thick protective horny layer in this area. Partial or asymmetrical patterns may be acceptable if related to close and repeated contact with irritants. But symmetrical vesicular palmar eczema alone is seldom primarily occupational. The feet should always be examined to exclude a fungal infection. Ingested allergens (even nickel and chromate in patients highly sensitive to these metals), heat, possibly stress and the atopic diathesis may be important in some cases. But the essential cause of this highly irritating and often explosive condition is unknown (see Chapter 8).

Finally, atopic dermatitis. Though probably less susceptible to delayed type sensitization, patients with the atopic diathesis appear to have a lowered resistance to irritants. Even those suffering from hay fever or asthma rather than eczema commonly show an intolerance to wool.

Children who have had atopic eczema when young and who are not advised about careers, may gravitate into engineering or hairdressing apprenticeships. In both these trades, they will be exposed to irritants and may not tolerate them. The result is an irritant dermatitis of the hands starting at any early age and which may be severe enough to prevent their finishing their apprenticeship. It is of great importance that all atopics should be counselled in early adolescence, before they become committed to unsuitable careers (Wilkinson 1975).

The course of atopic dermatitis is infinitely variable. The behaviour of the irritable skin is more subject than in ordinary people to the effects of heat and, probably, emotional upsets. Scratching further damages the skin and makes it more vulnerable to irritants. Therefore the pattern becomes complicated, and it is often extremely difficult to assess the role of occupational as opposed to other environmental factors in the behaviour of hand eczema (especially in this group of patients). The old adage, 'Would this have happened had he not been employed in this particular work?' often fails because of the concomitant effect of other environmental irritants at home or at play — for instance, soaps, detergents, gardening and so forth. One has to make the best assessment one can. Fortunately, most atopics learn what they are able to tolerate and what causes itching of the skin. Consciously or unconsciously, they usually adapt to this situation. But a latent atopic or one who has only had trouble in infancy but still is a constituted atopic may develop afresh an irritant-type dermatitis of the hands, either after marriage or childbirth, or when facing, however slightly, an increased contact irritant risk at work. It is in such cases that one faces difficulty in assessment. Although 17 of 93 patients with eczema were believed to be suffering from constitutional or general environmental exacerbations of their atopic state rather than from occupational causes, many who were accepted as having occupational dermatitis were, of course, atopic.

Summary

Remember — if you make a diagnosis of occupational dermatitis, a person's whole livelihood may be at stake and their future soured by concern, anxiety and litigation. Therefore observe the following points.

1 Be careful about initial certification. To a manual worker, 'dermatitis' means industrial dermatitis — not his fault and requiring compensation. To a doctor, of course, it may mean 'seborrhoeic', 'atopic', or 'neurodermatitis' but this is a subtle distinction for the person put off work because of it.

2 Always examine the patient's skin fully, at least on the occasion when you first make a diagnosis of an occupational dermatosis. Pay particular attention to the scalp, trunk and feet, but check also the state of the oral mucosa and the anogenital areas. More mistakes are made in dermatology by not looking than by not knowing.

3 When a patient presents with an eruption involving the hands, do try to note, in 'shorthand' if necessary, *what was the site* of initial involvement. If a civil claim for compensation is subsequently made, the medical assessors may be faced with a completely different picture and will need to have independent confirmation of the account given to them by the claimant, whose memory may be blurred by the passage of time. And do not forget to note whether your patient is left-handed. Not to know this, in a patient with a unilateral eruption, makes a lawyer's picnic!

4 Do not feel that you are losing the confidence of your patient (or yourself) by referring to a dermatologist anyone whose presumed occupational eruption lasts more than 2 weeks. The diagnosis and proof of occupational dermatitis is often extremely complex and difficult. The dermatologist will be able to obtain the exact nature of the substances regarded as the cause and he may well be seeing, at about the same time, other cases from the same factory. It was such a situation that led the author to set up the Industrial Skin Clinic; a small factory was on the point of closing because of the dermatitis caused by a new allergen. Each worker had a different doctor, and each worker was being taken off work, clearing and then returning to work into contact with the same allergen after clearing.

If waiting lists at the hospital are temporarily long, a personal telephone call to the dermatologist will probably enable your patient to be seen quickly. The dermatologist can also institute patch tests and can usually obtain the individual ingredients of a potential allergen which the worker has handled. This will enable an accurate confirmation or refutation of an allergic contact dermatitis to be made and the worker may then be reallocated to more suitable work, or avoidance techniques or substitution of the allergen may be attempted.

5 Do not forget that a manual worker incapacitated by dermatitis becomes anxious and insecure. He needs as much attention as someone who has lost a leg; he has 'lost' his hands. A dermatologist can only give guidance in treatment up to a limited point in the future. As the situation changes, so should the treatment.

6 Check that your patient, while off work, is not endangering his recovery by using soaps, helping in the house, or allowing any irritant to come in contact with his damaged skin. Counsel him to avoid shampooing his hair with bare hands and to avoid scrubbing his hands after gardening or painting. To the doctor, this may be obvious; to the patient, it is not.

7 Always try to keep in contact with the works' medical officer or, in cases of prolonged invalidity, the district regional officer. This is particularly important when the patient is young and has years of working capacity in front of him.

The GP is the lynch-pin, counsellor and permanent advisor of the patient. The industrial milieu is now so complex that all those with expertise should be involved round the GP, with the aim of curing the dermatitis and restoring the worker to the most gainful form of employment that the skin can tolerate.

References

Björnberg A. (1968) *Skin Reactions to Primary Irritants in Patients with Hand Eczema.* Oscar Isaacson, Göteborg.

Fisher A. A. (1973) *Contact Dermatitis*, 2nd edn. Lea & Febiger, Philadelphia.

Wilkinson D. S. (1975) Careers advice to youths with atopic dermatitis. *Contact Dermatitis*, **1**, 11–13.

Wilkinson D. S., Budden M. G. & Hambly E. (1980) A 10-year review of an industrial dermatitis clinic. *Contact Dermatitis*, **6**, 11–17.

- *The few specialist industrial dermatitis clinics have proved their value — more should be established.*
- *Many industrial sensitizers are also encountered in the home.*

Chapter 6
Primary Irritants and Solvents

W. A. D. GRIFFITHS & D. S. WILKINSON

Primary irritants are substances which, on contact with the skin, induce erythema and epidermal damage, producing a non-allergic eczematous response with limited exposure and a bullous reaction or necrosis with more intense exposure.

The range of potential skin irritants is unlimited and all chemicals, whether in solid, gaseous or liquid phase, must be regarded with suspicion and treated with caution.

Effects of irritants on the skin

Although the term 'irritant dermatitis' is commonly used for all types of inflammation resulting from irritants on the skin, this can be designated more accurately as listed below.

Subliminal irritant effects: no visible changes

Smarting occurs immediately in some people in reaction to a wide variety of substances including emollients and cosmetics that are tolerated by others.

Stinging. Also an idiosyncratic effect in people designated as 'stingers'. A more prolonged sensation occuring after a few minutes' contact. Antiperspirants containing aluminium salts may evoke it (Frosch & Kligman 1977).

These have few consequences in occupational terms.

The 'irritant reaction'

This is a very real entity and a useful concept. It consists of erythema, cracking, fissuring or 'chapping' — but not vesicle formation — occurring in response to a wide variety of irritants. It recovers within hours or days but tends to relapse quickly on further contact. It is one form of 'hairdresser's hands' and affects cleaners, housewives and others. Repeated attacks may lead to a true irritant dermatitis but it is not known what determines this.

True irritant dermatitis

There are three phases.

Acute. This always lasts longer, on removal from work, than the irritant reaction. But recovery is the rule.

Recurrent. With repeated attacks the recovery time becomes longer. Eventually it may pass into

Cumulative. Here the condition persists for a very long period, or is irreversible. The chronic machinist's or housewife's hand eczema are examples. It must be regarded as the result of a failure of control and care in the earliest phases. Malten's concept (see below) explains this situation.

Factors influencing the irritant reaction

A number of factors may interact with each other resulting in great variability in the precise pattern and degree of cutaneous reaction in any one individual.

Irritant factors relevant to the chemical

Nature of the chemical

Chemicals differ in their irritant properties on normal skin. Relative irritant potentials are not easy to determine because of the number of variables encountered in actual use. Various animal and human models have been proposed to predict irritancy of chemicals but no one system has emerged as completely satisfactory because of inconsistencies and frequent false negative results.

Concentration

In general, the more concentrated the chemical the more irritant it becomes but some chemicals may prove to have low irritancy even in high concentration.

pH

The greater the divergence of the chemical from the normal slightly acid pH of the skin — pH 5.6 ('acid mantle') — the more irritant it becomes. Continual exposure to substances of pH differing significantly from normal may alter the bacterial flora of the skin and thus add to the local effect by degrading chemicals in contact with the skin.

Temperature

Very hot or cold chemicals change the superficial cutaneous flow. Chemical interaction with the skin follows the normal rule of chemical reactions with a halving of the reaction time for each 10°C rise in temperature of the reagent.

Duration of exposure

The length of time an irritant remains in contact with the skin is a major determinant in the damage resulting. This may be relevant where a worker is doing an appreciable amount of overtime, or when an undetected hole in a rubber glove allows contact during much of a shift.

Frequency of exposure

That this is a key factor in the breakdown of skin has been recognized in recent years. Malten (1981) has emphasized that the effect of a repeated chemical or physical trauma on the skin is cumulative. In discussing the mechanism of irritant dermatitis, he has formulated the following proposition. There is an individual threshold at which a given subject will manifest signs of irritant dermatitis on exposure to an irritant of sufficient strength. Previous exposures may not have attained this threshold but make the skin more susceptible to further exposures. Eventually the threshold is breached and dermatitis appears. On discontinuing contact, it subsides but not always to the same 'base-line'. Each increment of exposure therefore leads to a quicker relapse. Eventually, the baseline exceeds the threshold and recovery does not take place.

Cumulative irritant dermatitis has occurred and created a situation that can only be very slowly, or not at all, irreversible.

This highly important principle of cumulative insult makes it easier to understand why it has been difficult to find an accurate and reproducible *in vivo* test for irritancy. Remember, also, in this context that the cumulative effect is non-specific. Changing a worker from one process in which he is experiencing skin trouble to another involving different irritants will not help with irritant dermatitis (cf. hypersensitivity allergic dermatitis).

We should also note the useful expression 'wear and tear' dermatitis (also called 'traumiterative'). This especially affects the palms, knuckles, forearms and finger pulps (with disappearance of the fingerprints). It is characterized by excessive dryness, desquamation, hyperkeratosis and fissuring; and by erythema at points of friction.

Physico-chemical interactions

The application of a chemical to the body surface initiates a series of reactions in the microenvironment, which include interaction with the surface sebum and the protein of the stratum corneum. The protective acid mantle of the skin may be altered. The whole of the intact stratum corneum acts as a barrier to the inward diffusion of chemicals through the skin, but skin appendages provide a natural, and chaps and fissures an easier, short cut to penetration. The effects of lipid solubility, partition coefficients and many other physico-chemical variables which influence percutaneous absorption have been extensively investigated by the pharmaceutical industry. Barry (1983) has provided a comprehensive review of these aspects.

Irritant factors relevant to the individual

Body site

The thin skin of the eyelids, the neck, scrotum and the antecubital fossae are more vulnerable to the effects of irritants than the thicker tougher skin of the palms or the back. If exposure is heavy in these sites several precautions may be taken. The period of exposure can be strictly limited, protective clothing such as goggles or apron may be provided or the process itself can be adapted to minimize exposure.

Ambient temperature and humidity

Both sweating and a high relative humidity increase hydration of the stratum corneum and enhance percutaneous absorption of chemicals. Occlusive protective clothing may exacerbate this further if chemicals get underneath through damage or incorrect use.

Constitutional weakness

Though definite evidence is still lacking, there is considerable support and some clear evidence for the view that the atopic subject is more prone than others to develop irritant dermatitis. In a group of young women hairdressing apprentices, Wilkinson & Hambly (1978) found that a previous history of atopy worsened the prognosis and that most such subjects abandoned hairdressing before completing their apprenticeship. Wilkinson (1975) suggested that atopic subjects should be steered away from work involving contact with wet irritants, especially hairdressing and manual engineering.

This lowered threshold for irritancy does not extend to allergic contact sensitization. In fact, this group is probably less at risk, except from medicaments, lanolin and preservatives in the topical applications that they have to use so frequently on their skin. It has been shown that atopics have a reduced capacity to bind water in their skin (Werner, Lindberg & Forslind 1982). This may be an important factor in their reactivity to irritants.

Career guidance at the age of 12–15 years for all those who have, or who have had atopic dermatitis, is a form of preventive medicine that should be endorsed by all GPs and school medical officers. Unfortunately each leaves it to the other.

There has been a widely held belief that the fair Celtic skin is much more susceptible to the effects of irritants than, for example, a Negro's skin. Two recent studies using dithranol as a standard irritant attempted to correlate irritancy with the fairness of skin classified according to the ease with which skin burns on exposure to ultraviolet light. These workers found no correlation between irritancy potential and the fairness of skin.

Conditioned hyper-irritability

This term has been given to a very important phenomenon in which the irritability of the 'normal' skin is heightened (or its threshold lowered) by the presence of eczema elsewhere on the body (Roper & Jones 1982). Thus a patch of eczema on the leg may lead to an irritant dermatitis developing on the hands of a worker who has previously tolerated the same industrial irritants. The patient may not recognize the importance of telling the doctor about the patch, since it may not seem to him to be related to his work, hence the importance of ***always examining the whole body*** of anyone presenting with a presumed irritant dermatitis of his hands. Lesions on the leg seem particularly prone to excite this reaction. Sometimes there is an associated medicament sensitization. Conversely, patients with hand eczema may react with a lowered threshold to irritants elsewhere. This can cause false interpretation of patch test reactions; investigations should therefore be delayed until the acute stage of eczema is past. The cause for this enhanced irritability is unknown but it appears to relate to cutaneous inflammation rather than to allergic mechanisms.

Worker compliance

Among any workforce there is a wide variation in the ability to understand risks and safety regulations, and in its willingness to comply with them. Case studies have repeatedly shown that a factory in one part of the country may have a persistent problem with a process which is apparently carried out safely in an identical manner in a factory elsewhere. Careful observation of the work actually being carried out is the only solution here. The use of barrier creams and gloves is considered elsewhere. An apparent relationship of a cutaneous problem to one particular work process may on closer examination turn out to be related to other factors. In one investigation of an outbreak of skin trouble among delivery men, the drivers were reluctant to handle one product produced by the firm, allegedly because of their previous experience of skin irritation when handling it. An important consideration, however, was that those drivers who were changed to another part of the roster were able more frequently to deliver another product to domestic clients — an operation which was easier and frequently attracted substantial tips.

Additional skin exposure

It has already been emphasized that the principle of cumulative insult is non-specific. Additional exposure of the skin to irritants encountered at home is frequently overlooked. The housewife with a young family, the man redecorating his home, repairing his car or gardening are exposed to additional quotas of skin damage. Second jobs of a part-time nature, so-called 'moonlighting', may be difficult to investigate and assess in relation to the main occupation. A clean skin may be praiseworthy, but soap and (especially) detergents do not help in the recovery of the damaged area.

Physical trauma

The role of mechanical, frictional, shearing and other forms of physical trauma to the skin has been underestimated. We know that fibreglass causes a positive irritant reaction as a result of penetration of spicules into the skin, but we ignore the effect of cuts, fissures, abrasions, and the microtrauma brought about by repetitive frictional effects — all of which destroy, to some extent, the integrity of the important stratum corneum barrier against penetration by irritants and sensitizers. Machinists working with swarf and even hairdressers in contact with the frictional effect of hair keratins may sustain repeated microtrauma to their skin, increasing the chance of irritant or sensitization dermatitis. Individual workers recovering from an irritant hand dermatitis should be warned against shampooing their hair. The combined effect of (concentrated) detergents and friction on their hands will impede recovery and may well worsen the condition.

Friction from repeated contact with wet reels of paper can cause an irritant dry fissured condition of the pulps of the first two or three fingers of the worker's hands. Newspaper deliverers handling the rough edges of papers on rounds in the winter may develop the same condition. Friction from tool handles, trowels or golf clubs can initiate a hyperkeratotic palmar dermatitis in managers and those retired, as well as in individual workers.

Common problems with industrial irritants

Some problem substances are so frequently encountered in industry that they merit further discussion here. Soluble oils are discussed in Chapter 7.

Soaps and detergents

It is a commonly held belief that soaps and detergents are strong irritants to the normal skin. This is not so. They are certainly effective degreasing agents and remove lipids temporarily with the dirt, but the human skin is very efficient in restoring this and in countering the effect of alkalinity or of many stronger irritants as used in everyday life. At times there are situations in which cleansing agents may damage the skin. Some soaps do appear to be more irritant than others when tested in an *in vitro* chamber test system. Frosch & Kligman (1979), who have made such an assessment, point out some situations in which this irritancy may become manifest. Winter chapping (irritant reaction) is often associated with over-washing (and incomplete drying). It recovers in even one day of moist warm weather, but if it continues it may allow other irritants to penetrate the disturbed protective horny layer or, in some cases, to become cumulative and an ingredient of housewive's dermatitis. They comment also that 'fanatical cleansing is common in those with diseased skin — the obsessional hand washers'. Dermatologists rightly advise alternative, bland cleansers in those with eczema. A few women with 'sensitive skin' cannot tolerate soap easily on the face or perhaps even in the bath — a sort of subliminal irritant reaction of 'intolerance', but this is sometimes due to a true allergic sensitivity to the perfume in the soap, rather than the soap itself.

Some of the bad reputation attached to detergents stems from old wives' tales and a fear of new technological achievements. Some is due just to bad housekeeping in using more than the recommended amount. 'If one shake is good, two shakes must be better', and again, a very few cases may be due to a true allergic sensitivity to perfumes, etc. It is very rare, in practice, to be able to demonstrate this as a specific primary cause of dermatitis.

Solvents

These are widespread in industry, of various types with varying capacities for irritancy. Though their prolonged use may cause an irritant dermatitis in any workers, older men are more likely to suffer, especially in the winter months. Even if not actively working with solvents, it is still unfortunately common practice to clean oil, paint or resin from the hands with petrol, paraffin or other solvents. It is not commonly recognized that some solvents easily penetrate rubber or PVC gloves, as shown by a rise in blood levels.

It must be stated that it is impossible to conceive of an ideal solvent. If it is to do its job of degreasing an object efficiently a solvent will inevitably degrease the skin and may lead to damage. Scrupulous care in handling solvents is essential and the deleterious effects can be minimized by regular use of an emollient preparation, such as Vaseline, Emulsifying Ointment or E45 cream, after a period of work. The non-cutaneous effects of solvents should also be remembered. For a detailed discussion, the reader is referred to the comprehensive monograph by Browning (1965).

Hand involvement

The hands are naturally the main area affected by occupational irritant dermatitis. In a recent review of some 340 cases of irritant dermatitis, they were involved in over 90% of cases. It is always taught that the backs of the hands and fingers and the interdigital spaces are predominantly affected because the palm is protected by its thicker skin. This was indeed so in these patients, but not exclusively. The backs of the hands and fingers were followed in frequency by the interdigital spaces and then by the palmar surfaces of the tips of the fingers (the pulps). Among substances and working processes causing this distribution were friction, paper handling, paper manufacture (roller 'feeling'), solvents, glues and household wet work. In contrast, hairdressers tend to have involvement of the backs of the knuckles.

The palms are not always spared and may, at times, be affected alone, especially the thenar eminences (see 'wear and tear' dermatitis above). But it is very rare for the *sides* of the fingers to be involved in irritant dermatitis.

Atopy and irritant dermatitis

Atopic subjects who have recently had, or who still have, atopic dermatitis are certainly more prone to irritant dermatitis; those who have had atopic eczema in the past are probably also more prone. These are the subjects whose skin breaks down on taking up unsuitable employment involving prolonged contact with irritants that are usually tolerated by others, e.g. hairdressing and machining.

The susceptibility of those with other atopic diseases, rhinitis and asthma for example, has not been sufficiently evaluated, but there is some evidence to suggest that they also may be at greater risk.

The 'dry skin' of the atopic is known to represent a subliminal atopic dermatitis and subjects with this are certainly more likely to develop an irritant dermatitis when in contact with irritants. How far this is attributable to their predisposition and how far to the working conditions is always a contentious medico-legal issue.

The common irritants

Wet work in general, particularly when carried out in conditions conducive to repetitive minor trauma, is the most common cause in women. Cleaners are at particular risk. The high incidence of nickel sensitivity found in hospital cleaners reflects both an increasing concentration of nickel in the buckets and cloths used and also the easier entry of allergens into a skin damaged by traumatic wet work. Thiuram sensitivity from the rubber gloves worn is a further risk.

Adolescent girls who become hairdressing apprentices or who do Saturday morning work are also vulnerable to irritant dermatitis from constant shampooing.

Other irritants, particularly affecting women, include any of the many household irritants that have still not been completely superseded by machines: lavatory cleansers, scouring powders, silver polish, etc. Detergents, if used in the correct dilution, are no more irritant than soaps to a normal skin; but they are often misused. When the skin is damaged it becomes more vulnerable to both irritants and allergens and it is hard for the housewife to prevent any form of hand eczema from becoming cumulative. Even shampooing the hair combines exposure to a degreasing agent with frictional trauma (see below). An irritant dermatitis of the tip of the third (long) finger has been caused by cleaning debris from the base of washing-up machines. Handling food may cause contact urticaria but also has an irritant effect, e.g. peeling potatoes or cutting onions or citrus fruit. Atopics seem to be particularly prone. Flour may act as an irritant in baking but is now more of a professional than a household risk.

Irritants from DIY activities are a common risk of both sexes, particularly since they are 'amateurs' and often fail to appreciate the degreasing effect of solvents in paints, etc. But non-manual workers have time to recover, whereas housewives have to continue to subject their hands to other household irritants.

Among men, the most common irritants that are involved in chronic cases coming to dermatologists are soluble oils and solvents (see Chapter 7). Solvents in paints are also implicated. The use of all these is often compounded by vigorous cleaning with white spirit, paraffin or other solvent-based cleansers. The number of other occupational irritants is legion; each trade carries its own risk — detergents and chapping in agricultural workers; chemicals in laboratory workers and the chemical industry generally; resins, glues, diesel oil, paraffin, acids and alkalis, etc. in a wide range of industries and occupations. Fibreglass is a well-recognized irritant giving rise to a characteristic clinical picture. Even the individual craftsman is not exempt (though he is usually a more careful and meticulous worker). But accidental spillage or breakage, e.g. of strong acids, may occur unexpectedly at any time.

Uncommon or unrecognized irritants

Bacterial toxins or exudates play an important role in many non-occupational skin diseases, e.g. around ileostomies, colostomies, leg ulcers and other orifices or damaged areas. In other situations, e.g. the flexures, intertriginous dermatitis or napkin erythema result from a combination of damp or sweat, friction and occlusion. Formaldehyde, ammonia and other fumes may cause a transient irritant erythema of the face. Those handling malt get 'maltster's itch'. Cardboard and paper dust may affect packers.

Friction and microtrauma

The role of friction in the causation of irritant dermatitis has been underestimated. It can be evident, as in those using abrasive materials, or it can be hidden and unappreciated. Repeated contact with hard swarf, metal dust or harsh powders causes damage to the stratum corneum which may be imperceptible but nevertheless sufficient to allow easier penetration of irritants and allergens. The housewife and most mechanical manual workers inevitably suffer repeated minor abrasions, which are visible but which do the same. The normal response to localized repeated friction is hyperkeratotic — a callus. But this does not form under the varied and changing exposure to friction cited above, particularly if the subject already has a slightly damaged skin. An executive noticed a slight but repeated 'dryness' and cracking of the pulps of some of his fingers and the webs after car washing in the winter. He then became a pig farmer and developed a more persistent palmar and interdigital hand eczema whenever he handled the pigs whose mobility ensured the maximal frictional effect from their bristles. Recently cases of pure frictional dermatitis have been reported from wire scouring pads and even from the (microscopically) rough surface of a table top. Friction is also an integral part of chapping (see below).

Climatic irritant factors

The chapping and desiccating effect of cold, dry winds is known to everyone. But its practical applications may be broader. The older factory worker who uses solvents and then washes with a degreasing agent and goes home with unprotected hands in winter conditions is subjecting his skin to repeated minor insults. Hot working conditions are uncomfortable and, in extreme forms, induce sweating with an increased tendency for dust irritation or flexural soreness, e.g. tunnellers. Heavy protective clothing may intensify the discomfort. Women who flush easily show this more markedly when coming in from the cold to the heat. Outdoor workers who have poor circulation or are inadequately clothed may develop erythrocyanosis of the legs or thighs or chilblains of the fingers, especially if carrying heavy objects.

Low humidity has been increasingly recognized as a cause of some 'constitutional' conditions, such as asteatotic and nummular eczema and as a cause of some occupational dermatoses, e.g. an itchy erythema of face and neck in employees in a soft lens manufacturing factory. This was cured by raising the ambient humidity from 30–35% to 45–50%. A low humidity, at the factory or in the house, should always be suspected in elderly workers with 'winter itch'.

Airline hostesses may suffer in a similar way; some have overcome it by spraying water on their faces with a perfume spray.

Prevention

The individual susceptibility to irritant dermatitis varies widely and even the best working conditions will not protect everyone as long as irritants are ubiquitous in most occupations and, indeed, in everyday life. But close attention to the following should greatly reduce the incidence.

Education and instruction

There is a widespread misconception that everyone knows about the behaviour of skin. This is not so. It is a very dynamic organ, subject to continued change, and though it normally has a superb defence mechanism, this does not extend to extremes of insult. The defences are breached by trauma or chapping, lowered by the presence of eczema elsewhere and by ageing. Workers handling any irritants should be taught the risks, not only by notices (which are often not read) but by personal instruction.

Early recognition

Not all those who develop irritant reactions go on to a cumulative irritant dermatitis; but they are certainly at risk of doing so. Early warnings should be taken seriously and treated appropriately.

Reduction of contact

Sometimes it is impossible to remove contact with irritants entirely, e.g. soluble oils in those working on moving machinery. But simple measures or a change in working methods are often possible to reduce contact with solvents, etc. Care, common sense and good housekeeping are essential and both the management and the worker himself must share this responsibility. If gloves are worn, they should be intact and of the right size and type for the work (see Chapter 9). Semi-automatic devices to reduce contact have not, perhaps, been sufficiently developed; perhaps not enough encouragement has been given.

Dirty and contaminated clothing must be changed frequently.

After-work measures

Workers using solvents are particularly in need of after-work emollient creams. Shower facilities are still a luxury but their value is unquestioned.

Time for restitution

Anyone who has suffered a chemical or thermal burn knows that the area remains highly reactive and irritable for many months. To a less extent this is also true of irritant dermatitis but here it is not recognized. Even when the skin has apparently returned to normal, it remains unstable and physiologically vulnerable for some weeks. Hence the common relapse very soon after return to work. When he does return, the worker should, ideally, be personally instructed in how to reduce or minimize contact with the particular irritants to which he is exposed. And he should continue to use creams and perhaps soap substitutes and avoid domestic irritants, such as hair shampooing, for several weeks more.

References

Barry B. W. (1983) *Dermatological Formulations*, Dekker, New York.

Browning E. (1965) *Toxicity and Metabolism of Industrial Solvents*. Elsevier, New York.

Frosch P. J. & Kligman A. M. (1977) A method for appraising the stinging capacity of topically applied substances. *Journal of the Society of Cosmetic Chemists*, **28**, 197–209.

Frosch P. J. & Kligman A. M. (1979) The soap chamber test. A new method of assessing the irritancy of soap. *Journal of the American Academy of Dermatology*, **1**, 35–41.

Malten K. E. (1981) Thoughts on irritant contact dermatitis. *Contact Dermatitis*, **7**, 238–247.

Roper S. S. & Jones H, E, (1982) A new look at conditioned hyper-irritability. *Journal of the American Academy of Dermatology*, **7**, 643–650.

Werner Y., Lindberg M. & Forslind B. (1982) The water binding capacity of stratum corneum in dry non-eczematous skin of atopic eczema. *Acta Dermato-Venereologica*, **62**, 334–336.

Wilkinson D. S. (1975) Careers advice to youths with atopic dermatitis. *Contact Dermatitis*, **1**, 11–13.

Wilkinson D. S. & Hambly E. M. (1978) Prognosis of hand eczema in hairdressing apprentices. *Contact Dermatitis*, **4**, 63.

- *Irritant reactions are much commoner than true sensitization.*
- *Fair skin is not more easily irritated than dark skin.*
- *Vulnerability to skin irritants lasts longer than clinical examination may suggest.*
- *All solvents are potentially hazardous to the skin.*

Chapter 7
Soluble Oil Dermatitis

R. RYCROFT

What is soluble oil?

'Soluble oil' is a misnomer since it consists of droplets of oil emulsified, rather than solubilized, in water. It is a convenient term because it is short and widely understood in British industry. It is one of the three different types of fluid that can be used industrially to lubricate and cool the machining (working) of metals and certain other hard materials such as glass (workpiece).

Metalworking, such as cutting or grinding, is carried out on high-speed machine tools. Without some form of cooling the cutting tools, which are commonly made of toughened steel or carbide, would be destroyed by the frictional heat evolved. Almost every manufactured product, whether metal or not, is made either with machine tools or with processing apparatus that itself has been made with machine tools. Metalworking fluids are therefore widely used. The other two types of metalworking fluid, besides soluble oil, are 'neat oils' and 'chemical solutions' (Table 7.1).

Neat oils are based usually on mineral oil, but may also contain animal, vegetable and synthetic oils. Their main additives contain

Table 7.1. A classification of metalworking fluids

Neat oils		Mineral, fatty or synthetic oils or combinations thereof. No water
Water-based metalworking fluids	Soluble oils	Oil-in-water emulsions of mineral, fatty or synthetic oils or combinations thereof
	Conventional	More than 50% oil in concentrate
	Semi-synthetic ('synthetic')	Less than 50% oil in concentrate
	Chemical solutions (synthetics)	Wetting agents, corrosion inhibitors, etc., in water. No oil

sulphur, chlorine or phosphorus, which improve the adherence of oil to metal surfaces under the pressure of the cutting tool (extreme pressure additives). There is no water in their formulation and they look like thinner versions of engine oil. Neat oil is often referred to by machine operatives as 'oil', 'mineral oil' or 'cutting oil'. Though soluble oils have partially replaced them, neat oils are still widely used. Neat oils are more likely to cause oil acne (folliculitis) than eczema. They were the main type of metalworking fluid associated with skin cancer. To remove carcinogenic polycyclic aromatic hydrocarbons, the mineral oil now used in them is solvent-refined instead of produced by straight distillation.

Chemical solutions or synthetics are the exact opposite of neat oils. They contain no oil but are solutions of wetting agents, corrosion inhibitors and other additives in water. A synthetic looks like water, though can be coloured, and may be referred to simply as 'water'. They are becoming increasingly used in place of soluble oils. Like soluble oil they tend to cause eczema rather than folliculitis.

Table 7.2. The main groups of soluble oil constituents

Mineral oils	Medium viscosity, solvent refined
Fatty oils	Animal, vegetable
Synthetic oils	e.g. polyalkylene glycols
Emulsifiers	Anionic, e.g. petroleum sulphonates, carboxylic acid soaps (some wood rosin derived)
	Non-ionic, e.g. ethoxylates
Corrosion inhibitors	e.g. sodium nitrite, triethanolamine, 2-mercaptobenzothiazole (MBT)
Extreme pressure additives	e.g. sulphur, chlorine and phosphorus compounds
Coupling agents	e.g. aliphatic alcohols, glycols, glycol ethers
Anti-foams	e.g. waxes and silicones
Perfumes	
Dyes	
Biocides	e.g. orthophenyl phenol, formaldehyde, formaldehyde-releasers such as hexahydro-1, 3, 5-tris (2-hydroxyethyl)-s-triazine (Grotan BK)

Soluble oils are supplied to factories as mixtures of oil, emulsifiers and other additives in drums (soluble oil concentrate) (Table 7.2). They are emulsified with water at the factory, in concentrate:water ratios usually between 1:5 and 1:50, to form milky fluids. These are commonly white, becoming grey or pale brown with use, but can be coloured with a dye. Their alkalinity usually ranges between pH 8 and 10. Soluble oil is also referred to in British factories as 'coolant', 'mystic', 'slurry', 'soup', 'suds' or, again, 'water'.

The concentrates of most 'conventional' soluble oils contain 50–80% solvent-refined mineral oil (Table 7.1). Those of 'semi-synthetic' soluble oils contain less than 50% mineral and/or fatty oil, their oily portion being supplemented by synthetic lubricants such as polyalkylene glycols. Semi-synthetic soluble oils currently account for only a small minority of the market in Britain. The other main component of a soluble oil concentrate, besides mineral oil, is a mixture of emulsifiers. These are commonly anionic with or without non-ionic additions (Table 7.2). In general, anionic emulsifiers are more aggressive to the skin than non-ionic, though anionics probably become less aggressive when mixed with non-ionics.

What skin problems can soluble oil cause?

Skin contact with soluble oil can cause an eczematous dermatitis, which may be termed soluble oil dermatitis. Oil acne (folliculitis) is not a problem with soluble oil. There are four characteristics of soluble oil dermatitis that require particular emphasis:

1 it is frequently patchy or discoid;
2 it is endemic more than sporadic;
3 it is most commonly a chronic irritant contact dermatitis;
4 susceptibility to it varies unpredictably between individuals.

Frequently patchy or discoid

The most characteristic pattern of soluble oil dermatitis on the skin is a patchy one, involving the forearms, the backs of the hands or the backs and sides of the fingers and the webs between them. Patches are frequently round or oval, attracting the terms discoid or nummular. Clinicians should therefore take care not to confuse this appearance with the discoid type of endogenous (constitutional) eczema.

Patchy patterns, though predominant, are not the only ones to be found in soluble oil dermatitis. Sometimes a continuous sheeted dermatitis can develop on the backs of the hands or on the forearms. Occasionally diffuse follicular eczemas are seen. Scaly finger webs are sometimes the only finding. Lichenified fissured dermatitis can become generalized over the backs of the fingers.

Why soluble oil dermatitis so often appears in small patches is not understood, but it is well recognized that chronic irritant contact dermatitis from other materials, such as cement and detergents, frequently takes on this same pattern.

Endemic more than sporadic

In a year-long study of over 100 machine operatives who had heavy skin contact with soluble oil in a ball-bearing factory, as many as a third of the workforce, and two thirds of new workers, were found to show some degree of soluble oil dermatitis at some time. Very few of these men were unable to continue in their jobs and even fewer lost any time from work. It is against such an endemic background of low grade dermatitis that sudden increases in prevalence ('outbreaks') may sometimes occur. It is usually difficult to find single causes for such outbreaks and a multifactorial aetiology should be considered (Table 7.3).

There may be reasons for sporadic rises in the irritancy of soluble oil emulsions that are not yet understood. Also the prevalence of soluble oil dermatitis has sometimes been observed to increase following the introduction of a workforce to an unfamiliar soluble oil or to a different factory environment. There may perhaps be a parallel here with the temporary surge of customer complaints that frequently follows the launch of a new cosmetic skin product. In each case the prevalence of complaints usually subsides without having to withdraw the new product.

Most commonly chronic irritant

Patch testing patients with soluble oil dermatitis can detect sensitization to certain constituents of soluble oil systems (Table 7.4)

Table 7.3. Some factors in the multifactorial aetiology of soluble oil dermatitis

Man	→ **Degree of skin contact with soluble oil***
Individual susceptibility	
Protective clothing	
Barrier cream	
Conditioning cream*	
Skin cleansers	
Systems of work and payment	
Work habits*	
Psycho-social*	
Unfamiliarity with machine type, soluble oil (in general/type/brand), or factory environment	
Machine	→ **Degree of skin contact with soluble oil***
Machine type	
Control method	
Fixed features of machine design	
Alterable features of machine design*	
Ease of cleaning sump mechanically	
Soluble oil	
Chronic irritancy of emulsifiers	
Wetting and drying cycles	
Alkalinity	
Mechanical trauma from metal particles	
Soluble oil type	
Strength of emulsion*	
Length in use*	
Contact sensitizers (see Table 7.4)	
Biocide addition in use*	
Deterioration in use from physical, chemical and biological factors	
General	
General factory environment*	
Climate	

Bold lettering denotes proposed importance.
* Those factors usually most amenable to useful change in a given factory.

and should therefore be carried out in persistent cases. False negative results can be obtained with used soluble oil emulsions and false positive results with unused soluble oil concentrates. Patch testing should therefore be carried out by a dermatologist trained and experienced in the technique.

Patch testing is most often negative and when sensitizers are detected there is usually an important chronic irritant component

Table 7.4. The best documented contact sensitizers present in water-based metalworking fluid systems

Balsam of Peru
1, 2-Benzisothiazolin-3-one (Proxel)
1-H Benzotriazole
Chromate (added/leached out)
Cobalt (leached out)
Nickel (leached out)
Colophony (wood rosin)
Dichlorophene (Panacide)
Ethylene diamine (Proxel CRL)
Ethylene glycol
Formaldehyde
Hexahydro-1, 3, 5-tris (2-hydroxyethyl)-s-triazine (Grotan BK)
2-Hydroxy-methyl-amino-ethanol-tri-N-ethyl-hydroxy-2-amino-methylene (Forcide 78)
2-Mercaptobenzothiazole
N-Methylol-chloracetamide (Grotan HD, Parmetol K50)
Pine oil
Triethanolamine

Many are weak sensitizers, especially at the concentration used in soluble oils, and should not necessarily be excluded from use because of their presence in this list.

to the dermatitis in addition to sensitization. A change of soluble oil to one no longer containing the relevant sensitizer may improve the soluble oil dermatitis but rarely clears it. The dermatitis of patch test-positive patients looks very similar to that of patch test-negative patients. Sensitization may therefore be a secondary event rather than the primary cause. It remains important to detect since continuing contact with a sensitizer will prevent the spontaneous recovery that often occurs in purely irritant soluble oil dermatitis.

The emulsifier content of soluble oils is arguably the most significant factor inducing skin irritancy over prolonged periods. Alkalinity, oil and suspended metal particles may play supporting roles.

Levels of the sensitizing metals chromium, cobalt and nickel have been shown to rise while a soluble oil is in use, but only under special circumstances have particularly high levels been detected. It is unlikely that levels sufficient to cause significant sensitization are present in the majority of machining operations.

Simultaneous investigations of the bacterial flora of a soluble oil in use and of the skins of machine operatives heavily exposed to that soluble oil have shown no evidence that bacteria in soluble oil emulsions colonize the skin and initiate or maintain soluble oil dermatitis. The considerable metabolic activity of the soluble oil microflora leaves open the possibility that some of its metabolic products may act as skin irritants, or even sensitizers, and that soluble oil micro-organisms may thus indirectly contribute to dermatitis.

Susceptibility varied but unpredictable

In the year-long epidemiological study previously referred to, machine operatives with similarly heavy soluble oil contact varied from complete resistance to dermatitis to high susceptibility. No clinical features could be found which would reliably predict susceptibility, with the probable exception of a strong personal history of atopic eczema.

This lack of predictability argues for the close surveillance of large occupational groups working with soluble oil. Only in this way can susceptible individuals be identified early; they should then be given every chance to continue in their work before a permanent job change is advised.

The liberal use of emollients (skin conditioning creams — see Appendix 2) and the regular application of a dilute fluorinated topical steroid may allow a mild irritant dermatitis to recover while contact with soluble oil continues. If this fails then soluble oil contact should be avoided until the dermatitis is clinically clear. This usually takes 1–2 weeks. If at all practicable a transfer to dry work is far preferable to time off work altogether. If dermatitis begins to recur on return to soluble oil contact, once again a chance should be given for clearance on treatment while work continues. If this is unsuccessful then a prolonged period of 2–3 months away from soluble oil contact is worth a trial, to allow more than simply clinical recovery to take place. By this stage patch testing should be carried out as comprehensively as possible. If patch tests are negative and industrial hygiene optimal but subsequent return to soluble oil contact is followed by unmanageable relapse then a permanent transfer away from soluble oil contact is usually the best medical advice. Even then the author has seen such advice steadfastly rejected and full recovery eventually occur.

How can soluble oil dermatitis be prevented?

It must be accepted that among large numbers of machine operatives heavily exposed to soluble oil, a small degree of low grade dermatitis probably cannot be prevented. The prevention of a higher prevalence of more severe soluble oil dermatitis can be considered from three aspects: the person, the machine and the soluble oil.

The person

Those with personal histories of long-standing atopic eczema, particularly if it involves the hands or forearms, should at the very least be warned of the potential of soluble oil to aggravate their eczema. Unless very strongly motivated indeed, they would be well advised not to embark on the type of engineering work where long-term heavy soluble oil contact is likely. Operators and setters of production machinery tend to have much heavier contact with soluble oil than toolmakers.

Gloves are usually ruled out because of the danger of their being caught up in rapidly revolving machinery. Some of the more automatic machines may allow the wearing of gloves and impermeable sleeves (armlets) would appear to be less dangerous than gloves. A major problem with such protective clothing is that of soluble oil entering the open ends of gloves or armlets and then being occluded against the skin. Also gloves easily become lacerated, often only minutely, by sharp fragments of metal and may then let in soluble oil over a long period before the wearer realizes. Occlusion of soluble oil against the skin will enhance its irritancy.

Barrier creams tend rapidly to be removed by the emulsifier content of soluble oils. The liberal and thorough application of a water-repellent barrier cream may allow sufficient to adhere throughout a working shift to facilitate subsequent skin cleaning. Milder skin cleaning agents can then be used at the end of the shift. In this way barrier creams probably can make some contribution to preserving the integrity of the epidermis, which may otherwise be threatened by more aggressive skin cleansers. If a way can be found of inducing soluble oil workers to apply an emollient cream routinely after washing, better preservation of epidermal hydration following skin cleaning would be expected and some enhancement of resistance to soluble oil dermatitis might result. The difficulty lies in achieving such routine usage before, rather than after, the onset of dermatitis.

Systems of work and bonus payment of a workforce and the work habits of individuals may encourage increased amounts of soluble oil contact. The industrial medical officer may detect such influences by close observation. It should not be forgotten also that the general environment of a factory can deeply affect employees' morale and attitudes and that these psycho-social factors can influence greatly the employees' response to a dermatitis problem among them.

The machine

The machine tools which recur with the greatest regularity in the histories of patients with soluble oil dermatitis are those that result in the highest degree of skin exposure to soluble oil. It is impossible to give accurate ratings of relative risk to different machine types because the total number of employees working on each type of machine is not known. However, the machine tools which recur with the greatest frequency in London are manually fed capstan lathes, manually fed vertical drills and multispindle automatic lathes.

Manual feeding of workpieces, lack of instantaneous cut-off of soluble oil flow when cutting tools are withdrawn before adjustments and a need to steady the workpiece with one hand under the flow of soluble oil are three of the main factors which significantly increase the degree of soluble oil contact and thus make dermatitis more likely. A machine tool on which soluble oil may be used as the metalworking fluid should ideally be designed in such a way that it can be run with the minimum need for contact between soluble oil and the skin of its operatives. Numerically controlled (NC) and fully computerized machine tools are the best solution but are still not widely enough used in Britain to have made much impact. Their increasing use should reduce the prevalence of soluble oil dermatitis in the future.

Other machine characteristics which increase the degree of skin contact with soluble oil include: a frequent need for manual workpiece changing or tool changing and adjustments; a need to make more than one type or size of workpiece on the same production machine; a frequent need for checking workpieces for size and quality; lack of reliability of machinery calling for frequent repairs; the closeness of parts needing frequent adjustment to the ends of pipes delivering soluble oil to the machining area of a machine; high machining speeds increasing splashing and decreasing tool life; a frequent need for removal of metal fragments (swarf) from the machining area. It is worthwhile for industrial medical officers to look for machine features such as these; and transfer of an operative with soluble oil dermatitis from a machine with many such features to another with fewer, and hence less soluble oil exposure, may assist recovery.

The soluble oil

With conventional soluble oils commanding such a large share of the market in Britain, it is difficult to draw any firm conclusions as to whether other types of water-based metalworking fluid are more or less likely to cause dermatitis. If it is correct to assign to emulsifiers a leading role in the irritancy of soluble oils, then semi-synthetic soluble oils, with their greater excess of emulsifier over oil than conventional soluble oils, might be expected to be more irritant to the skin than conventional soluble oils, and wholly synthetic chemical solutions to be potentially even more irritant.

Balancing anionic emulsifiers with higher percentages of non-ionic emulsifiers, or even excluding anionics altogether in favour of non-ionics, are the formulation changes that might have the highest potential for decreasing the irritant potential of conventional soluble oils. Technical considerations at present make this difficult to achieve. Choice of the type of crude mineral oil used in refining oil for soluble oil concentrates might also have some influence though the evidence for this is less firm.

At present there is still no generally agreed and reliable test procedure for assessing the chronic skin irritancy of materials such as soluble oil emulsions. Until there is such a test, a vital part of the primary prevention of soluble oil dermatitis is lacking.

It is part of sound prevention to use the least sensitizing technically effective additives in soluble oil formulations and to use them at the lowest technically effective concentration. Low concentrations may in fact allow the use of chemicals, such as formaldehyde and 2-mercaptobenzothiazole (MBT), that *a priori* would appear likely to cause sensitization problems. Care must be taken not to overemphasize the potential harm of additives of known sensitizing abilities used in very low concentrations, for fear of encouraging the use of theoretically safer alternatives which in practice are sometimes found to be worse than the original.

It is sound policy never to introduce a new soluble oil to a factory without first informing the workforce and consulting the industrial medical officer. When a soluble oil change with inadequate consultation is followed by an increased dermatitis problem, quite understandable feelings of resentment can arise among operatives and the industrial medical officer may quite justifiably consider himself to have been excluded from a decision with important bearings on the future health of his patients.

Allowing the strength of soluble oil emulsions to rise uncontrollably as water evaporates appears to increase the likelihood of dermatitis. In general, the weaker the emulsion the weaker are its potentially irritant constituents likely to be and the less irritant the emulsion to the skin. Engineering considerations demand a certain minimum strength. A compromise must therefore be achieved between engineering and dermatological demands. Regular checking of emulsion strength is recommended from both points of view, either in a quality control laboratory or with a refractometer on the shopfloor.

It is less certain whether soluble oil emulsions become inherently more irritant with use, excluding this concentration effect. In factories with soluble oil dermatitis problems, increasing the frequency of complete soluble oil changing and sump cleaning has appeared to help decrease the prevalence of soluble oil dermatitis. It is difficult to place much reliance on this impression, however, since factories never make just this one change in isolation in response to a dermatitis problem. Allowing soluble oil emulsions to lie stagnant in sumps for days or weeks on end would seem particularly to encourage microbial deterioration and perhaps thereby increase the risk of irritancy.

Extreme overdosing of soluble oil emulsions with additional

biocides in use can increase their irritancy by over-increasing their pH. The use of additional biocides on the shopfloor should be both rational and adequately monitored. Their usefulness in the prevention of dermatitis is often overestimated.

The future

The greater the proportion of computerized machine tools in British industry the smaller the problem of soluble oil dermatitis is likely to become. Meanwhile industrial medical officers, GPs and dermatologists can all do much to foster a better understanding within the engineering industry of the skin problems associated with soluble oils. Advance in our understanding will depend on co-ordination between the scientific, technical and medical investigation of the problem. Further research is particularly needed into the variation in individual susceptibility to soluble oil dermatitis and the relative skin irritancy of different soluble oil emulsifier systems.

- *Soluble oil dermatitis may mimic some constitutional eczemas.*
- *Soluble oils may contain additives with a risk of sensitizing the skin.*

Chapter 8
Hand Eczema in Industry and the Home

R. CHURCH

The site where dermatitis begins (through trauma or sensitization) is the point where the causative irritant is most strongly concentrated. It follows therefore that, both in industry and the home, the hands are the commonest area affected. In both instances the most frequent cause is trauma, which implies that the hands have been exposed to an irritant substance in sufficient concentration for long enough for it to damage a normal skin. Whereas in industry most work processes are sufficiently circumscribed for the likely causes of dermatitis to be pinpointed in any one case, in the home the possible contacts are legion and it is likely that traumatic dermatitis at least is multifactorial.

History

When one is confronted with a patient with eczema of the hands, a good and accurate history is the most likely way to reveal the cause.

Where?

If due to external causes the dermatitis should have started on the hands at a time when the rest of the skin was normal. If there were already lesions elsewhere then, unless the hands had been protected with gloves, it is worth considering other diagnoses, e.g. if the feet were first affected, tinea pedis with cheiropompholyx; if the flexures of the limbs, atopic eczema; if elbows and knees, psoriasis.

When?

In industry the eruption should have started when the employee was at work, as opposed to on holiday or off work for some other reason. For any particular job to be incriminated, the eczema should have started for the first time while the employee was doing that work. Possibly it may have improved at weekends or when on holiday. In the case of the housewife it should have started when she started this work; previous skin trouble on the hands while still at school suggests atopic eczema.

Why?

A detailed account of the way the job is carried out, what substances are encountered in the work and what protection is used, especially gloves, may reveal an obvious cause of skin irritation. If the same work has been done for years with previous impunity it is possible that there has been a change in the substances encountered, such as addition of bactericide to a coolant oil.

In the case of the housewife, the arrival of the firstborn increases exposure to soap and detergents and causes the change in work which precipitates dermatitis.

Alternatively the work may be clean, dry and innocuous and the family history of eczema, asthma and hay fever suggest that the case is one of atopic eczema.

Examination

Examination will reveal whether the eruption on the hands is eczematous or else some disease such as psoriasis which is unrelated to occupation. A search of the rest of the skin will also exclude other possible causes of an eczematous eruption on the hands such as tinea pedis, a leg ulcer or widespread nummular (discoid) eczema.

In theory, the distribution of dermatitis over the hands should be an aid in diagnosis: external contacts, both traumatic and sensitizing, tend primarily to affect the thinner skin on the dorsum of the hands and the webs of the fingers, while involvement of the palmar aspects with sparing of the dorsum suggests an endogenous cause, except in the rare cases where the sensitizer is an implement held in the palm. In practice this convenient rule may be broken, so that sometimes traumatic dermatitis mainly affects the palms and allergic dermatitis may produce the appearance of a constitutional pompholyx on the palms.

Rings on the fingers trap irritants under them and are often the initial site of traumatic dermatitis in the housewife. Involvement of the tips of the fingers may suggest some sensitizing substance such as resin glues and the classical cause, the rubber finger stall, is occasionally seen. Although dermatitis is often worse on the right hand (in right-handed people) it is uncommon for one hand to be completely spared; if in such a case the palm and finger nails are involved the diagnosis is more likely to be a fungus infection with Trichophyton rubrum. The nails may be pitted and opaque in psoriasis, but it is also usual for the nail plates to become transversely ridged and possibly pitted on those fingers which are involved in chronic dermatitis.

Having established that the patient is suffering from an eczematous eruption on the hands, which the history suggests is occupational, it is a matter of attempting to define the cause which may be trauma or sensitization.

Industrial dermatitis

Traumatic or primary irritant dermatitis

In the diagnosis of a primary irritant dermatitis one is dependent on the history, as patch tests are only of value in allergic contact dermatitis. Skin tests for irritants have been devised, but they are difficult to interpret and have not yet been standardized.

The common causes of traumatic dermatitis of the hands in industry are acids, alkalis, detergents and degreasing agents. When the subject has been found to have had constant exposure to these substances at work without the protection of gloves they are most likely to be the cause of dermatitis, though when sensitizers have also been encountered it may be necessary to exclude them by patch testing.

Acids

In strong concentrations these cause burns, but hydrofluoric acid is sometimes used in dilute form as a cleansing agent and causes erythema of the unprotected hands.

Alkalis

These also cause burns in strong concentrations but in lower concentrations cause dermatitis. Sodium hydroxide is present in cleaning agents and disinfectants and in using these the hands should be protected with gloves.

Soluble oils normally have a pH of 8–9 but errors in its dilution or sometimes the actual addition of sodium hydroxide as a rust preventive may make it much more alkaline. Many of the engineering processes in which these oils are used, drilling, milling, etc., make the wearing of gloves hazardous and hands wet with an alkaline solution all day eventually develop dermatitis. In recent years, cutting fluids containing little or no oil have been increasingly used; these contain sodium nitrite which is a primary irritant and their pH is 8–10.

The fact that wet cement is strongly alkaline is responsible for its ability to produce alkali burns and skin necrosis in those unwise enough to kneel in it for prolonged periods. It has a more chronic effect on the skin of the hands producing a low grade fissured dermatitis and nail dystrophy.

Degreasing agents

Fat solvents, of which trichlorethylene is the best known, are used to remove grease and dirt in numerous engineering, plating and electrical apparatus manufacturing processes. These solvents obviously remove fats from the skin just as efficiently, yet it is still possible to encounter workers using these substances on rag wipers without wearing gloves. Even when gloves are provided they need to be chosen with care as it has been shown that they penetrate most types of gloves and especially PVC.

Detergents

Excessive exposure to detergents also removes surface fats from the skin, and its occupational effects outside the home are most frequently seen in hairdressing apprentices, who often spend most of the time in their first year shampooing hair. Of those who develop dermatitis of the hands, over half acquire this within the first year of their work, and the high incidence of sensitivity to hair dyes in these girls is probably due to the predisposition to become sensitized when suffering from a traumatic dermatitis of the hands. Cleaners are the other large group at risk from detergents and among these can be singled out home-helps employed by local councils who go from one house to another using whatever detergents are available, frequently being careless about the use of gloves (see Chapter 6).

Sensitization dermatitis in industry

A study of occupational dermatitis in five European skin departments showed that in a standard battery of tests chromates and rubber chemicals produced a higher number of positive reactions in those with occupational as opposed to non-occupational dermatitis.

Cement

In many countries dermatitis in building workers is responsible for between 20 and 30% of all occupational dermatoses. In over half of those with a cement-induced eczema the hands and arms are involved, and 74% of these are found to have a positive patch test to chromate. It is the hexavalent chromium, soluble in an alkaline environment, that causes sensitization. Addition of ferrous sulphate to the cement reduces the chromate to the insoluble trivalent form and in Scandinavian countries is being used to render the cement less harmful. The appearance of cement dermatitis on the hands may misleadingly resemble a constitutional pompholyx.

Coolant fluids

While an irritant dermatitis is the commonest result of exposure to coolants they also contain numerous potential sensitizers. Antioxidants present in some oils which are recorded as having caused sensitization are aromatic amines, phenolic compounds and mercaptobenzthiazole. Bactericides such as Grotan BK and Panacide CA have been responsible for outbreaks of sensitization dermatitis and soluble oils also contain dyes such as fluorescein and perfumes which are potential sensitizers. As if all this was not enough, the hardened steels which are worked nowadays contain nickel, chrome and cobalt. Salts of these metals are formed during the machining of these alloys. The levels reached are unlikely to cause sensitization dermatitis.

In carrying out patch tests to soluble oils it must be remembered that the additives are present in such low concentrations that if the oil is used in the working dilution no reaction will be obtained. It should therefore be used neat and at 50% in olive oil. If positive reactions occur, it is a wise precaution to test the constituents further and separately.

Rubber

There are numerous accelerators, anti-oxidants and other chemicals contained in synthetic rubber which make it a common cause of industrial dermatitis of the hands. Rubber gloves are an obvious hazard when worn to protect the hands, but also those who handle car tyres, cables, rubber tubes and rubber bands may develop dermatitis of the hands. In the case of those handling car tyres, the dermatitis tends to affect the palms, especially the thenar eminences, where it produces redness, scaling and fissuring.

Epoxy resins

Synthetic resins have become a common cause of dermatitis in recent years and of these the occupational risks from epoxy resins are the highest. Aircraft, car and paint factories, and the electrical and electronic industries are the most likely areas for industrial contact. On the fingers a subacute papulo-vesicular eruption is commonly seen but it is usual for the eyelids to be affected at the same time.

Dermatitis in the home

The term housewives' dermatitis was at one time synonymous with a traumatic dermatitis of the hands caused by primary irritants such as soap and soda. Modern detergents have taken the place of these substances. However, in most cases it is probably due to multiple factors of wet work and detergents, household cleaners and disinfectants plus the traumatic effect of handling food such as flour dough. The common time for dermatitis to develop is after the birth of the firstborn when nappy washing adds one more insult to a skin on the verge of breaking down.

Sensitization dermatitis

The possible substances encountered by a housewife which could cause a sensitization dermatitis are so numerous that the results of battery patch testing are more helpful here than in industry in drawing attention to an unsuspected cause.

In a survey carried out in five European clinics (Calnan *et al.* 1970) of a series of 4000 patients, 281 were women engaged in domestic work only who were suffering from contact dermatitis of the hands. These were all patch tested to a battery of substances similar to that recounted below which is used at St John's Hospital London. Just over half (53%) had a positive reaction to at least one substance. The allergens responsible occurred in the following proportions: balsams 27%, nickel 14%, medicaments 10%, cobalt 8%, rubber 7%, chromates 5%, benzocaine 5% and paraphenylenediamine 5%.

A similar number of housewives with contact dermatitis of the hands was studied by Agrup who considered that 38% were allergic and the rest irritant; in her and other surveys nickel sensitivity had the highest incidence.

A standard battery is given in Table 8.1. The relevance of these patch tests is given by quoting the number against some common causes of dermatitis. Full details are given in Appendix 3.

Rubber gloves (Battery 13, 3, 11, 17)

Ironically rubber gloves worn to protect the hands, sometimes because traumatic dermatitis has already developed, are one of the commonest causes of sensitization dermatitis in the housewife. The area of the hands involved often shows sharp upper edges at the border of the gloves on the wrists. If rubber gloves are worn a square cut from a glove should be added to the battery patch test.

Table 8.1. A standard battery

1	Potassium dichromate
2	p-Phenylene diamine
3	Thiuram mix
4	Neomycin sulphate
5	Cobalt chloride
6	Benzocaine
7	Nickel sulphate
8	Quinoline mix
9	Colophony
10	Parabens
11	PPD mix
12	Wool alcohols
13	Mercapto mix
14	Epoxy resin
15	Balsam of Peru
16	p-Tertiary butylphenol formaldehyde resin
17	Carba mix
18	Formaldehyde
19	Fragrance mix
20	Ethylene diamine dihydrochloride
21	Quaternium 15
22	Primin

For full details, see Appendix 3.

Nickel and cobalt (Battery 7, 5)

Despite the fact that suspenders have been unfashionable in recent years, nickel sensitivity remains very common in women, the allergy probably being acquired from cheap jewellery and clothing clips. Once acquired, it is almost impossible to avoid handling nickel-containing metals in the home and the sensitivity is often associated with sensitivity to cobalt.

Nickel plating may be present on needles, pins and cutlery, while stainless steel, much used for kitchen equipment, cutlery and scissors, has been shown to release nickel when exposed to sweat and detergents. Nickel-containing metals can usually be demonstrated by the dimethylglyoxime test. Hand eczema has been shown to occur in about half the nickel-sensitive women and conversely about one-fifth of women with hand eczema are nickel-sensitive. Hand eczema in these nickel-sensitive women is frequently of the pompholyx pattern — producing tiny vesicles on the palms and the sides of the fingers. The first thing to eliminate is continuing contact with nickel in clothing clips and ornaments, and it is often extremely difficult to get this necessity across to the patient.

In those with enough intelligence to have eliminated external contact with nickel, continuing hand eczema can be due to ingestion and a low nickel diet has been used with variable results. In essence this consists of avoiding tinned foods and acid foods cooked in stainless steel utensils, certain vegetables and fruits, tea and chocolate.

Flour

Baker's dermatitis can, of course, also be found in the housewife. The degreasing effect of the sticky dough plus the use of cleaning materials make an irritant dermatitis the commonest. However, in Great Britain, ammonium persulphate and benzoyl peroxide are added to flour as 'improvers' and both can give rise to a contact urticaria or a sensitization dermatitis.

Foods

Allergic reactions to the handling of foods are uncommon. The most well known is sensitivity to garlic and onions which produces dermatitis on the finger tips similar to that found in bulb growers and known as 'tulip fingers'. It is common for this to affect one hand only — that holding the clove or onion while it is chopped.

Carrots can give rise to both an allergic and an irritant dermatitis and although usually limited to the hands of those scraping carrots, it can spread to other exposed areas. Of the same family is celery, which can produce an acute papulo-vesicular dermatitis on the hands and forearms. It is not handled enough to affect the housewife often but is a hazard in canning celery especially if it is handled when wet.

Fish and shellfish can cause eczema of the hands and have been incriminated as a common cause of dermatitis in Danish sandwich makers. In some cases patch tests are positive, in others scratch tests, and in some a positive patch test can only be obtained by applying it to the previously involved skin.

Balsams (15)

The high incidence of sensitivity to balsams in both housewives and in male workers with eczema of the hands is probably due to the fact that both groups encounter these in perfumed soaps and hand creams. In addition, the housewife encounters these substances in the spices and flavouring agents used in cooking, those most commonly causing dermatitis being capsicum, cinnamon, cloves, nutmeg and vanilla.

Parabens (10)

The esters of p-hydroxybenzoic acid are so widely used as preservatives in cosmetics, foods and medicaments that the incidence of sensitivity is small. However, the common source of contact in a hand eczema would be the creams being applied for treatment and these should be reviewed if the battery test reveals this sensitivity.

Plants (22)

The housewife is often a very poor witness as to whether she has plants in the home. If she can remember having them she usually has no idea of their names, but if she was given a pink-flowered plant for Mothers' Day it was probably a *Primula obconica* which is the commonest cause of non-occupational plant dermatitis in Europe. This causes blistered areas on the fingers where the leaves have been touched in picking off dead ones. The blisters dry and desquamate in a few days only to reappear elsewhere. An additional clue is given by the appearance of blistered streaks on the forearms, neck or face where the fingers contaminated by the leaves have touched.

Sensitivity to other plants such as chrysanthemums or tomatoes is more often seen in the person who keeps a greenhouse and usually extends to other exposed areas.

Resins (14)

The finding that many women give a positive reaction to patch tests with epoxy resin is a reflection of the extent to which these substances are used in the home. Uncured epoxy resins are used in the manufacture of other plastics and handling domestic articles made of PVC has produced dermatitis of the hands. (See also page 36.)

Prevention

The most effective measure of prevention in both industry and the home is to keep the hands out of contact with irritants and sensitizers; in the factory automation has achieved this in many work processes, and in the home clothes-washing machines, dishwashers and electric floor cleaners must have been responsible for the undoubted drop in incidence of dermatitis. In processes which still have to be performed manually, gloves provide considerable protection, though it is often difficult to avoid contaminating the inside if they are doffed at intervals. The housewife should be encouraged to use lined PVC gloves in preference to rubber. In the factory, gloves need to be chosen with care to be appropriate for the job; it should be obvious that for wet work impermeable gloves are necessary, yet it is not unusual to see workmen issued with cotton-backed gloves to protect them against soluble oil. It has been shown that acrylic monomer and nickel salts will pass through thin rubber gloves and that various solvents penetrate most types of glove, polyvinyl chloride being the most easily penetrated, and neoprene and nitrites providing the best protection. It is not possible to wear gloves for certain mechanical processes in engineering because of the hazard of trapping them and the hand.

The idea that creams applied to the hands could form a barrier which would prevent dermatitis has been current for several decades. It has been shown experimentally that cutting oil penetrates such creams in about 3 minutes, this being in static conditions and not those of work where the hands are moving and are exposed to an intermittent stream of coolant fluid. It has also been argued that 'barrier creams' facilitate hand cleansing at the end of the shift. This has been tested by assessing the removal by washing of a mixture of grease and soot applied at the end of the shift when barrier cream had been used at the beginning. Although there were minor advantages in favour of the barrier cream these disappeared when a slightly more effective cleanser was used. Most dermatologists now accept that barrier creams perform little useful function, and in addition they may cause active harm, as those with an unusual fat content can increase absorption of aniline compounds, and the oil-resistant creams, which contain soap, when used under occlusive gloves can actually cause dermatitis.

For those who cannot wear gloves, cleanliness, education and conditioning creams are the best protection. Factories now have to adhere to the Factories Act (1961) which requires that adequate and suitable facilities for washing shall be provided for the use of employed persons, which should include a supply of clean running hot and cold or warm water and, in addition, soap and clean towels or other suitable means of cleaning and drying; these facilities shall be conveniently accessible and shall be kept in a clean orderly condition.

Education is a matter of warning those who are handling potential irritants and sensitizers of the dangers and how they may be minimized. The 1974 Health and Safety at Work Act now makes it obligatory for employers to inform the employees of these risks.

Conditioning creams applied at the end of the shift are better known to the housewife than the workman but they could be used with advantage in the factory (assuming that they did not increase the already high fragrance sensitivity!).

Prognosis

In theory, if the cause of hand eczema can be identified and removed recovery should be swift. In practice the outlook is extremely variable and depends on the duration of disease before receiving expert attention, whether it is an irritant dermatitis or sensitization and, if the latter, how easy it is to avoid the allergen.

In a study of hand eczema (Wilkinson *et al.* 1970), 25% of the patients, both male and female, had suffered from the condition for over 5 years, yet, after testing, 26% of another series (Agrup 1969) had recovered completely within 6–26 months.

Where traumatic dermatitis is concerned it is certainly one's impression that rapid removal from the cause of the trouble, for example in young hairdressers, is usually followed by complete recovery, yet in the case of housewives with traumatic dermatitis, often long established before they seek expert help, the condition seems to grumble on indefinitely despite their efforts to avoid irritants.

Allergic contact dermatitis due to substances which can be completely avoided characteristically improves rapidly, so that the workman may notice that his hands even improve at weekends only to relapse on return to work. Allergens such as nickel and chrome, however, are ubiquitous and once dermatitis of the hands has occurred in nickel-sensitive patients it may be extremely difficult to clear it because of its presence not only in plated articles but also in numerous alloys, so that even 7 carat gold may contain appreciable quantities of nickel depending on the source.

Sensitivity to chromate is more common in men and usually occupational. It has been shown that this particular sensitivity has a worse prognosis than sensitization to other allergens. Cement dermatitis has in the past been thought to have a very poor prognosis, yet it has been shown that even those who have become chromate-sensitive can make a complete recovery while still working with cement and that a significant number of cement workers who have changed their job because of cement dermatitis have continued to have trouble with their skin. The difficulties likely to be encountered by a manual worker in finding alternative employment make it advisable for him to be encouraged to continue at work keeping his dermatitis at bay with gloves and treatment in the hope that it will in time improve or even clear.

Management

The manual worker and the housewife readily conclude that their eczema of the hands is caused by their work. For the worker, to receive compensation for this is of little comfort if he is out of a job as a result. It is therefore important to be as sure as possible about the cause before recommending any change in employment. In the case of the housewife, the job is lifelong, but her dermatitis is usually traumatic and advice about avoiding irritants by the use of gloves and, if possible, domestic machinery is often enough to control the trouble. Rubber gloves tend to make the hands sweat and may also sensitize, so either cotton gloves should be worn underneath or lined PVC gloves used.

The manual worker suffering from traumatic dermatitis can also often get the skin better if gloves can be worn for the job; if they cannot, a temporary move to other work may be enough to control the eruption and he may then be able to resume the original work, probably taking more care to protect his hands and remaining well, although traumatic dermatitis if already long established is liable to become chronic. In the case of sensitization dermatitis removal of the cause is more likely to be followed by a swift and complete recovery than is traumatic dermatitis, and when sensitization has been proved most workers so suffering must be moved from this contact otherwise there will be a steady worsening of the skin condition.

When dermatitis has occurred and the man is still at work, the way in which he is treating his skin needs looking into. The soapless cleansers and abrasive cleansers used in industry are almost certainly too harsh for an eczematous skin and he should be advised to take his own soap for washing. It is common for the ambulance room attendant in the factory to hand out a barrier cream to the dermatitis sufferer. The fact that in theory this should have been used to prevent rather than treat the dermatitis is of little moment for, as has already been remarked, its preventive properties are negligible; on the other hand, the oil-resistant barrier creams contain soaps which are most likely to add insult to the existing injury.

Treatment

In this country and in America there has been a drop in the incidence of industrial dermatitis by about 20% in the past 20 years (see p. 8). Much of this is due to improved conditions of work, but some is due to the rapid and effective treatment of early lesions with local corticosteroids. Dermatitis of the hands still becomes chronic in some cases and behaves like an endogenous eczema but the frequency with which this happens is slight compared with the days when tar paste was the only remedy. The skin of the palms has a thickened corneal layer which is less readily penetrated by corticosteroids than other areas, the hydrocortisones do little to control eczema in this site and it is preferable to use a fluorinated steroid application. Because of the tendency to crack round the knuckles an ointment is preferred unless the greasiness interferes with paperwork, when the cream base is preferable. Local corticosteroids should be applied twice daily. In the acute stages of dermatitis secondary infection can be a problem, the hands almost overnight becoming covered with vesicles and pustules accompanied by oedema. In such cases a systemic antibiotic should be given and wet dressings of Eusol or 0.5% silver nitrate lotion applied until the infection is overcome. When vesiculation subsides a corticosteroid–antibiotic mixture such as Propaderm-A ointment can be substituted. The chronic stages of dermatitis are more of a problem; the cause may have been removed, the worker may have sick leave but still the eczema persists or fluctuates. In such cases the use of Lassar's paste with tar at night applied under cotton gloves and cleaned off in the morning with liquid paraffin before reverting to corticosteroids in the day can control the eruption. Corticosteroid ointments penetrate the thickened keratin of the hands poorly, and if ordinary application twice daily produces no improvement it is worth advising the patient to apply the ointment at night and make the hand airtight under a disposable polythene glove, continuing this each night until the skin is virtually healed then using the ointment without occlusion. Instructions to keep the hands out of detergents are often followed only haphazardly by the housewife, and if lack of progress suggests this, the hands can be occluded under Coltapaste bandages for a week at a time until they recover. Those using an ointment base and still washing their hands should be given advice about soap, Simple soap or Neutrogena soap probably being safe to use, or emulsifying ointment can be used with advantage as a substitute for soap except when the hands are very dirty.

In those cases in which a fluctuating eczema still persists despite apparent withdrawal of external cause, superficial X-ray therapy, gray (100 rads) repeated fortnightly to a total of 3 grays (300 rads), is often a successful last resort.

Rehabilitation

Resettlement of a worker who has had to give up his job because of development of dermatitis of the hands is a thorny problem. In fortunate cases, the firm for which he works is able to find him alternative employment, but in others there may be no jobs in that particular firm which are free from potential dermatitis risk and he is forced to seek work elsewhere. In these circumstances it seems to do him an actual disservice to put his name on the disabled persons register, as he is branded for life as a dermatitis sufferer and few employers will risk taking him on. In times of normal employment, most workers who have any drive and incentive manage to find alternative work for themselves. Those with dermatitis who are ultimately put through rehabilitation courses to teach them other skills do not have a high success rate.

References and further reading

Agrup G. (1969) Hand eczema. *Acta Dermato-Venereologica*, **49** (Suppl. 61), 44.
Calnan C. D., Bandmann H. J. *et al.* (1970) Hand dermatitis in housewives. *British Journal of Dermatology*, **82**, 543.
Cronin E. (1980) *Contact Dermatitis*. Churchill Livingstone, London.
Fisher A. A. (1973) *Contact Dermatitis*, 2nd edn. Lea & Febiger, Philadelphia.
Wilkinson D. S. *et al.* (1970) The role of contact allergy in hand eczema. *Transactions of the St John's Hospital Dermatological Society*, **56**, 19.

- *The hands are commonly affected in both constitutional and industrial skin disease.*
- *Avoidance of specific sensitizers does not always lead to a cure.*
- *Fluorinated steroids may be indicated for palms, but beware of the dorsal surfaces of the hands.*

Chapter 9
Protective Gloves

D. S. WILKINSON

The need to provide industrial workers with adequate protective gloves is generally recognized and indeed stressed by contributors in this book. This is particularly important when potentially dangerous chemicals are being handled. The notes that follow in no way lessen the responsibility for their provision. But, like barrier creams, it is sometimes assumed that such gloves provide a perfect 'protective skin', and that merely to order the wearing of gloves is enough by itself to ensure the safety of the worker. This is not necessarily so. As with all safety devices, their value may be limited by practical or physical considerations; sometimes a compromise is necessary. The following points deal with some limitations which should be recognized.

Physical danger

The danger of trauma from the use of protective gloves when dealing with moving machinery is well recognized in industry and limits their use among most machinists.

Precaution. When essential, they should be close-fitting. Low tear strength Neoprene or Nitrile gloves are probably safer, as well as being resistant to cutting oils.

Splashing

Chemicals, oils or solvents may splash over the cuffs of gloves and run down under them — often not noticed by worker.

Precaution. Longer gauntlet-type; turn cuff back or tuck cuff under sleeves; or provide plastic sleevelets.

Minipuncture

May occur when used in handling sharp metal edges or tools,

though frank tears are more common. May be unobserved by worker.

Precautions. Frequent change of gloves. Test by water inflation and pressure. Both these events may cause a quasi-occluded effect of an irritant concealed beneath the glove and greatly enhance its effect.

Contamination

The outside of gloves may become grossly contaminated. This can be transferred to the skin by the fingers in pulling the gloves on and off, especially if this is done frequently in the course of a shift.

Precautions. Wash gloves before removing. Learn surgical 'no-touch' technique with turned-back cuffs. Do not leave gloves on a bench with chemicals or irritants with the cuffs turned back.

Sweating and discomfort

Many workers (and housewives) dislike wearing rubber or PVC gloves for any length of time, especially if they have sweaty hands. They find them uncomfortable and this may impose a psychological and physiological barrier to effective work performance. This situation becomes more marked if they suffer from cheiropompholyx or sweat profusely in the summer months or in hot working conditions.

Precautions. Relief can be gained by removing the gloves at regular intervals. In an industrial environment, it may be difficult to regulate this. Cotton-lined gloves may be helpful for short periods.

Penetration and permeation (Table 9.1)

It is now widely recognized that many chemicals are capable of penetrating rubber gloves, some rapidly and some only slowly or after the gloves have been 'injured' by wear or weakened by prolonged heating and soaking. Thin gloves are obviously more vulnerable. Substances capable of penetrating rubber and PVC gloves are discussed in Chapter 2. We have also shown penetration by a tiling glue. Detectable amounts of benzene and chlorinated

Table 9.1. Penetration through gloves (extracted from various reports)

Penetrant	Type
Acrylic monomer	Surgical rubber
Paint stripper	Natural rubber Neoprene Nitrile PVC *Not* PVA
Methanol	PVA *Not* normal rubber Neoprene Nitrile PVC
Nickel	Standard rubber
Dichromate	Surgical) Standard) rubbers *Not* 'heavy duty'
Tiling glue in solvent	Standard rubber
Formaldehyde 37%	Standard

solvents rapidly penetrate virtually all types of rubber polymer and PVC gloves. Viton gloves (Dupont Company) are impermeable but very expensive. However, they are mandatory in the United States for workers handling these particular groups of substances.

Precautions. PVC gloves are generally impervious and therefore safer for nickel-sensitive housewives with hand eczema. The London Rubber Company is very knowledgeable in this field and is always willing to advise.

Deformation and disintegration

Certain types of gloves are more suitable than others for those handling particular chemicals and, particularly, solvents. Workers may complain that their gloves become hard and stiff, or 'tacky' after some hours' use handling such materials.

Precautions. No perfect solution exists but a wide variety of synthetic gloves are now available and guidelines for a suitable

Table 9.2 Suitability of various protective gloves (extracted from *Glove Resistance Chart*, published by The London Rubber Company, LRC Products Ltd., North Circular Road, London E4 8QA)

Agents	Preferable gloves	Unsuitable gloves
Inorganic acids*	Neoprene, PVC Heavyweight rubber	Lightweight rubber
Organic acids (most)*	Heavyweight rubber Neoprene Nitrile	Lightweight rubber
Aliphatic solvents†	Nitrile Neoprene (some)	Rubber
Aromatic solvents	Nitrile (fair)	Most types
Chlorinated solvents	Nitrile‡	Most types
Vegetable oils	Nitrile, PVC Neoprene	Lightweight rubber
Soaps and detergents	PVC, Neoprene (Nitrile) Heavyweight rubber	Light and medium-weight rather less effective

* Consult *Glove Resistance Chart* for individual acids.
† Consult *Glove Resistance Chart* for individual solvents.
‡ Splash protection only.

choice are readily available from the London Rubber Company and other responsible bodies (Table 9.2). The worker must be provided with the type of glove most suitable for the type of work on which he is engaged and it is the duty of the medical safety or personnel officers to see that, as far as is reasonably possible, a correct choice has been made and that such gloves are available to the workforce.

Sensitization

Anti-oxidants and accelerators used in the manufacture of rubber gloves are potential sensitizers and may either cause an allergic contact dermatitis or perpetuate a pre-existing hand eczema by penetration of the allergen through broken skin. In this case the pattern usually changes to one uniformly involving the backs of the fingers and hands to a sharp 'cut-off' point at the wrists and forearms. The most common offenders are the chemicals belonging to the 'thiuram' group or dithiocarbamates. (A thiuram mix is a standard allergen in all patch test batteries.) Thiurams are responsible for about 15–20% of all positive patch tests in housewives, cleaners and domestic workers with hand eczema. Patch testing with a 1 cm square of new, uncontaminated glove is usually, but not invariably, positive. Both inner and outer sides should be tested since the rubber chemicals are often different at these sites.

Precautions. A change to PVC or other synthetic gloves is usually sufficient. Some rubber gloves are free of thiurams.

General references

The *Glove Resistance Chart*, published by The London Rubber Company, LRC Products Ltd, North Circular Road, London E4 8QA, provides much indispensible information and should be in the possession of all those dealing with industrial protection and safety and of medical officers concerned with workers at risk of contracting, or who have contracted, dermatitis.

The same firm has also produce a *Fact Sheet No. 1* (October 1980) and a comprehensive *Marigold Industrial Glove Catalogue* (ref. No. 1002). They have a wealth of information and an excellent information service available to factory managers and doctors.

Russell-Fell R. (1982) Hand in glove with rubber. *Protection*, **19/4**, 8. Published by A. Osborne, 22 Nelson Road, London SE14.

Lloyd G. A. (1976) *The Resistance of Air-impermeable Protective Clothing Materials to Penetration by Liquid Chemicals.* Operator Protection Group Report PC/1. Ministry of Agriculture, Fisheries and Food, Harpenden. This contains detailed studies of penetration by pesticides and their solvents and other related chemicals. Reprints in short supply; photocopies obtainable but chargeable. However, much of the information is contained in:

Lloyd G. A. (1979) Developments in personal protection. In *Proceedings of the 1979 British Crop Protection Conference — Pests and Diseases*, pp. 821–831.

The author would like to acknowledge the help given in the preparation of this section by Mr R. Russell-Fell, Technical Service Manager, LRC Products Ltd, while emphasizing that the responsibility for its contents is entirely that of the author.

- *Protective gloves may make some dermatoses worse through their occlusive properties.*
- *Sensitization to rubber may obscure an underlying dermatosis of different aetiology.*

Chapter 10
Barrier Creams

E. CRONIN

As long ago as 1915, R. Prosser White wrote that it is 'necessary that men's clothes and skin should be protected by overalls and suitable covering. Any cutaneous surfaces that have become soiled should be cleansed as soon as possible. To assist in this, some bland, insoluble ointment has been advised to be rubbed into the exposed surfaces prior to work. The quantity used should not be large, but enough to block up the stomata of the skin.' Thus started the search for a 'barrier cream' which would protect the skin by forming a film through which irritants, sensitizers and other toxic substances could not pass. Schwartz in 1942 did not place much reliance on the efficacy of protective ointments but thought that they should be available to be used by workers. He divided the protective ointments into six types according to their function:

1 to facilitate washing;
2 to form a thin film which, acting as an invisible glove, would help to protect the skin from irritants;
3 to protect the skin by filling the hair follicles and sweat ducts with a harmless fat;
4 to contain a harmless chemical which would neutralize toxic chemicals;
5 to coat the skin with a protective inert powder;
6 to protect against photodermatoses and from the phototoxic effect of tars.

The choice of the name 'barrier cream' was most advantageous in that this description of itself implies a benefit to the user, and simply by being called barrier creams, these preparations have been guaranteed a success which seems to have little basis in experimental evidence.

Manufacturers make many different types of barrier creams, advising that the correct barrier cream be used for different sorts of work and for the many different chemical hazards. Despite these many formulations, barrier creams are basically made for dry work and are then water-soluble. If they are intended for wet work, they must be water-insoluble, otherwise they would be washed off. The dry work creams may contain polyethylene glycols and those for wet work are based on paraffin and silicones. If the cream is to protect against acids or alkalis then it may contain organic buffers. More recently, all-purpose creams have been introduced which are designed to protect against every hazard. All these formulations aim to prevent degreasing of the skin, and with this object barrier creams are now often sold in conjunction with special skin cleansers intended to prevent workers from using harmful solvents or strong detergents for cleaning their hands and skin.

Since their introduction, there has been a slow trickle of reports in the literature concerning barrier creams, but few have substantiated the claim that they are able to protect the skin from either sensitisers or from irritants. Over the past 20 years there has been surprisingly little published for or against their use. To clarify the evidence the reports have been divided into those relating to sensitizers and those relating to irritants.

Sensitizers

Two early reports are a judgment of the effect of barrier creams on the shop floor. In 1963 and 1966, Engel & Calnan studied two outbreaks of dermatitis in a car factory, one from chromate in a primer paint, and the second from para-tertiary butylphenol formaldehyde resin in an adhesive. In both outbreaks about two-thirds of the men had used barrier creams, but these had done nothing to protect them from sensitization either to the chromate or to the para-tertiary butylphenol formaldehyde resin.

In 1971, Wahlberg described work done in the guinea-pig. He used radioactive chromate made up as an 0.4% aqueous solution and assessed four barrier preparations, two proprietary barrier creams, a silicone liquid and petrolatum. The creams were rubbed well into the guinea-pig's skin and the silicone liquid was pipetted on to the surface. The chromate solution was applied either 1 minute later or after 15 minutes. This 15-minute interval was selected as an estimate of the time between a worker applying the barrier cream and starting his work. Absorption of the labelled chromate was measured with a scintillation counter and a decrease in activity on the skin surface was a measure of the amount of chromate absorbed. Wahlberg found that a film of 1 mm thickness had to be reached before there was a detectable inhibition of the absorption of the chromate solution. Increasing the thickness of the cream gave less rather than more protection because a thickened layer of barrier cream actually facilitated absorption of the chromate. Wahlberg suggested that this was due to the barrier cream acting as a vehicle for the chromate and it then facilitated rather than hindered penetration.

Fischer & Rystedt (1983) studied the effect of barrier creams on patch test results in cobalt-sensitive subjects. To the subjects' skin they applied layers of barrier creams about 0.1 mm thick which they estimated to be double the thickness of that which would be used in practice. The patients were then patch tested over these layers of barrier creams with dilutions of cobalt chloride. It was found that the barrier creams offered no protection from the cobalt and, in fact, it was thought that they enhanced the patch test reactions.

Irritants

The evidence relating to irritants is of great importance, and there has been experimental work in man and guinea-pigs and also an evaluation of their effect on the shop floor. The efficacy of these creams to protect against the penetration of solvents has been assessed by measuring the excretion of the solvent in the breath of exposed subjects. This method was used by Guillemin *et al.* (1974) in Lausanne. Ten male volunteers immersed their hands in a container of toluene for 10 minutes with and without using one of two barrier creams. The subjects wore masks to prevent inhalation of the solvent. The overall results suggested that if the creams were carefully applied and rubbed well into the skin, then they did impede absorption of the toluene. In a further study, Lauwerys *et al.* (1978) utilized the same experimental procedure but used *m*-xylene as the solvent. They immersed their subjects' hands for 20 minutes and then measured the excretion of *m*-xylene in the breath and also the excretion of its metabolite, methylhippuric acid, in the urine. There were 13 volunteers and they used two barrier creams, one containing 10% silicone and the other glycerol and stearates. The initial estimations were the absorption of xylene through the skin of the unprotected hands, and in eight subjects the experiment was repeated to assess the variability in absorption at different times in one person. The absorption of xylene was then estimated after applying a barrier cream to the hands. It was found that xylene could be detected in the breath of a subject 10 minutes after the beginning of exposure, and the peak concentration was reached at 30 minutes, which was 10 minutes after the exposure had ceased. In one subject there was some variation in the amount of xylene absorbed from one exposure to another, but there was a much greater variation between individuals. Application of either of the two barrier creams to the hands before immersion in the xylene had no effect on its absorption through the skin.

In further work with solvents, Bohman, Wahlberg & Johansson (1982) used closed containers to apply toluene and benzene to guinea-pig skin and then monitored absorption by measuring the concentrations of the solvent in the guinea-pig's blood. Two hours after the application of toluene, the blood levels were the same for normal skin, skin protected by a glove or skin protected by a barrier cream. Similar results were obtained with benzene: both the gloves and the barrier creams had some initial benefit but were of no long-term help.

Lauwerys *et al.* (1980) have reported a study in which workers were exposed to dimethyl formamide in an acrylic fibre factory. They estimated absorption by measuring N-methylformamide in the urine. In workers wearing no protective clothing, the amount of dimethyl formamide absorbed through the skin is about double that inhaled by the lungs. It was found that long-sleeved gloves gave much greater protection to the workers than either of the two barrier creams investigated.

In their study, Fischer & Rystedt (1983) used barrier creams to assess a sparing effect on the skin from patch tests with dilutions of sodium lauryl sulphate, but as with cobalt the barrier creams gave no protection.

In clinical practice patch tests with barrier creams may give slight irritant reactions. Occasionally, barrier creams sensitize, the usual allergens being a preservative, a perfume or sometimes lanolin or one of its derivatives.

For the proper assessment of the value of barrier creams, closely supervised factory trials with and without barrier creams are required, but it is impossible to imagine such trials being undertaken. As yet a definite protective value for barrier creams has still to be proven.

References

Boman A., Wahlberg J. E. & Johansson G. (1982) A method for the study of the effect of barrier creams and protective gloves on the percutaneous absorption of solvents. *Dermatologica*, **164**, 157–160.

Engel H. O. & Calnan C. D. (1963) Chromate dermatitis from paint. *British Journal of Industrial Medicine*, **20**, 192–198.

Engel H. O. & Calnan C. D. (1966) Resin dermatitis in a car factory. *British Journal of Industrial Medicine*, **23**, 62–66.

Fischer T. & Rystedt I. (1983) Skin protection against ionized cobalt and sodium lauryl sulphate with barrier creams. *Contact Dermatitis*, **9**, 125–130.

Guillemin M., Murset J. C., Lab M. & Riquez J. (1974) Simple method to determine the efficiency of a cream used for skin protection against solvents. *British Journal of Industrial Medicine*, **31**, 310–316.

Lauwerys R. R., Dath T., Lachapelle J.-M., Buchet J.-P. & Roels H. (1978) The influence of two barrier creams on the percutaneous absorption of m-xylene in man. *Journal of Occupational Medicine*, **20**, 17–20.

Lauwerys R. R., Kivits A., Lhoir M., Rigolet P., Houbeau D., Buchet J. P. & Roels H. A. (1980) Biological surveillance of workers exposed to dimethylformamide and the influence of skin protection on its percutaneous absorption. *International Archives of Occupational and Environmental Health*, **45**, 189–203.

Schwartz L. (1942) Protective ointments and industrial cleansers. *Medical Clinics of North America*, **26**, 1195–1212.

Wahlberg J. (1971) Absorption — inhibiting effect of barrier creams. *Berufsdermatosen*, **19**, 197–207.

White R. P. (1915) *Occupational Affections of the Skin*, 1st edn, p. 94. H. K. Lewis, London.

- *The use of barrier creams may engender a false sense of security.*

Chapter 11
Causes of Unexpected Persistence of an Occupational Dermatitis

D. S. WILKINSON

All doctors dealing with patients with occupational dermatoses are only too well aware of the cases that do not clear up after removal from the original contact and supposed cause of the eruption, even with a reasonable period of sick leave. Sometimes this leads to extremely prolonged periods of absence from work, and causes increasing anxiety, litigation and disruption of the worker's social and family life. Such cases are commonly regarded as having changed into a 'constitutional eczema'. Some patients do, indeed, appear to develop a change of pattern of their disease or, after several attempts to return to work, a cumulative and chronic eczematous state (see Chapter 6, p. 61). We know little of the mechanism of eczema. In some cases a contact 'trigger factor' fires off a more protracted constitutional eczematous condition. But we tend to hide our ignorance of this situation without thinking of possible alternative reasons for the continuation of a primary occupational dermatitis. Such alternative causes must be diligently sought, since they are often wrongly dismissed as merely examples of this constitutional behaviour of the eczematous process. Insufficient attention is paid to many recognizable factors that may cause such chronicity or lack of response to supposedly adequate treatment during a period of sick leave. Some of these are discussed in this chapter.

Re-exposure at work

This is, of course, the most common cause of the persistence, exacerbation or relapse of an occupational dermatitis. It is not easy to avoid, particularly if there is only a limited scope in a given factory for a skilled worker, trained in one particular field. There are three ways in which this may happen. The first is the most common. Once a worker's dermatitis appears to be better, or even to have cleared completely, perhaps after only a short period off work, he is 'signed off' as being fit for work. Now, it is the obvious desire both of the doctor and of the worker that he should return to work as soon possible. There is also a prevalent fashion to believe in early rehabilitation — a swing of the pendulum from the days of protracted convalescence in many spheres of medicine. But visual, or 'anatomical' restitution of apparent normality of the skin is not paralleled by its functional recovery. Water loss through the stratum corneum has been shown convincingly to lag behind apparent recovery by several weeks (Malten 1981). Therefore the worker who returns to contact with an agent that provoked the initial dermatitis may be at a disadvantage in returning to this contact immediately after the stage of apparent visual recovery. A 'probationary' period of dry work is seldom possible (though it should be requested); a more prolonged period of sick leave will not easily be accepted by the patient unless the reason is explained to him; even then, with incredulity or disbelief, or an urgent need to recoup his financial losses. The best solution is probably to spend a little time explaining the continuing vulnerability of the patient's skin to him and to discuss what measures he can sensibly take to improve his standards of good housekeeping 'at work'; and to discuss the situation with the factory doctor or personnel manager. A second and subsequent breakdowns usually lead to more prolonged periods of invalidism and, eventually, a cumulative and perhaps irreversible dermatitis.

Cross-reaction

The second cause lies in unexpected and unforeseen cross-reaction in sensitization. A man working with epoxy resin developed an acute epoxy allergic dermatitis. His firm, acting in his supposed best interests, moved him away from the epoxy-mixing area but to one in which he was, unfortunately, exposed to contact with a solvent containing epichlorhydrin, a cross-reactor with epoxy resins. The employees did not know that this was incorporated in the solvent. He relapsed.

Degree of sensitivity

The high degree of sensitivity to epoxide diluent fumes is often not recognized. Even walking through an area where these are being used, on the way to the canteen for instance, may cause a relapse of a worker's dermatitis. This constitutes the third risk — that of inadvertent re-exposure due to unforeseen circumstances. A good factory doctor should be aware of this possibility and make sure that workers involved avoid such risks.

'Moonlighting'

Gainfully employed workers may be rather unwilling to disclose that they are undertaking other work 'outside hours'. Tact is necessary to elicit this information but it is sometimes of great importance. It is a more common practice than is recognized but chiefly affects men, since women regard whatever work they do outside the home as being their own form of extra income.

A young engineer developed an irritant dermatitis of his hands which improved greatly on a short period of sick leave. On his return to work, it was found possible to put him on to a relatively dry job using machinery without oil. But his condition relapsed and, indeed, spread and he was again off work, this time for several weeks. Only after patch testing revealed a positive reaction to dichromate did he admit that he had been engaged in the evenings 'helping' some friends, using cement for landscape gardening.

Unexpected patch test reactions, in particular, should alert the doctor to the possibility of such a hidden source of allergic dermatitis. But persistence of an irritant dermatitis due to a secondary occupation are harder to detect.

Hobbies

With increased leisure and technology, hobbies and occupational pursuits at home have become more diverse in recent years. Though any hobby can be considered as a 'mini-occupation' carrying, theoretically at least, the same risks, they are seldom the cause of irritant dermatitis in those with healthy skins. Probably a man is more fastidious about his hobby than about his work; certainly the conditions are less arduous, the hours shorter and the conditions cleaner. But workers, taking advantage of sick leave to extend their hobbies, may inadvertently perpetuate a dermatitis at a time when rest from work should bring about its resolution. 'Messing about in boats' may cause chafing, frictional damage and climatic insults; 'messing about with cars' involves contact with oil, petrol and hand cleansers. Fishing, golf, and darts may seem to carry no important hazards but allergic reactions to handle grips may, rarely, be the cause of persistent hand or finger eczema. Television viewing may affect those with long-wave light sensitivity. Woodworking, model-making or carpentry may involve some risk with glues or trauma, but DIY painting and decorating carries greater hazards.

Some hobbies are quite bizarre and may involve contact with sensitizers that have not been recognized as the cause of a man's original occupational dermatitis. As an intrinsic part of his environment, the hobby cannot be disregarded as a possible cause of perpetuation of an occupational dermatitis.

Infection

Any chronic eczema may become infected by the patient's own staphylococcal or by extraneous staphylococci and streptococci. Eczematous subjects are particularly good 'culture media'. Severe infective episodes such as cellulitis are easy enough to recognize. But a more insidious staphylococcal infection may complicate any occupational dermatitis or produce a secondary eczematous pattern of its own.

A man of 45 had developed a proven sensitivity from epoxy resins. After two relapses from return to working in proximity to the resins, he was moved to another part of the factory. But he continued to show a persisting pustulovesicular eruption of the palms and some discoid patches on the arms. These cleared after a course of antibiotics and when the strong steroid cream he was using was changed to a weaker one containing an antibacterial agent.

Suspect superinfection when:

- pustules or crusted lesions are present;
- there is any other source of infection in the patient;
- the worker has been using a potent topical steroid without the expected result.

Fungal infection

An active *Trichophyton* infection of the feet can give rise to a persistent or recurring 'ide' eruption of the hands, showing as a vesicular eczema of the palms or sides of the fingers ('pompholyx'). This is bilateral and roughly symmetrical and is more common in the summer months or under hot working conditions, especially when wellingtons or heavy duty boots are worn. It is recognized as an occupational disease of miners but this is partly because of the communal use of pithead baths. When a change of pattern occurs in a pre-existing dermatitis of the hands, the feet should always be examined and any plantar or interdigital fungus infection treated. Remember that fungal spores may remain viable for a year or more in shoes, socks and carpeted bathrooms. So bedroom slippers should be changed and prophylaxis counselled after apparent cure has been achieved.

A man of 56 had suffered a true exogenous dermatitis of the backs of the hands and fingers. His job was changed and for some weeks he remained fairly clear. But he began to complain of itching of the palms and sides of the fingers. This was attributed to a relapse and he was again taken off work, this time for some months. Subsequent examination of his feet revealed an active infection with *Trichophyton mentagrophytes* which he had not thought worth mentioning. Effective treatment of this allowed his return to work.

Persistent *unilateral* scaling of one hand may be due entirely to an infection by *T. rubrum* (which may be difficult to demonstrate microscopically). The feet are almost always similarly affected, though the scaling may be slight and easily overlooked.

Suspect fungal infection when:

- the pattern is one of 'pompholyx';
- it occurs or is worse in hot conditions;
- there is (usually unilateral) scaling, vesicles or erythema of sole or interdigital spaces of the toes;
- the toe nails are thickened, with yellowish-brown discoloration and linear streaking.

Household irritants and sensitizers

Though this hazard particularly applies to women, men who are unemployed may decide to try to do more to help in the house. Their speciality is probably painting and decorating, but gardening,

Table 11.1. Some household irritants and sensitizers

Irritants	Sensitizers
Sink and pan scourers	Perfumed substances
Lavatory cleansers	Rubber gloves
Soaps and detergents (in excess)	Nickel objects
Oven cleansers	Chromates in paints, etc.
Solvents, especially white spirit, paraffin	Epoxy resins
Heavy clay soils	Pot plants
Low humidity (flow heaters)	'Strike anywhere' matches
	Formaldehyde and formalin releasers
	Black rubber (hoses, etc.)
	Over-the-counter topical medicaments
	Garden insecticides

Table 11.2. Simple precautions to be taken in the home

Use soap substitutes (emulsifying ointment or similar bases) for affected areas
Protect hands when shampooing
Wear leather or cotton gloves when gardening
Avoid excessively hot water
Make full use of mops and 'no-touch' techniques
Do not use perfumed creams
Wear plastic, not rubber, gloves
Use emollients if your skin is dry

washing up and cementing may also be undertaken. They may not appreciate that, even when away from a causative agent at work, they have a damaged skin with a reduced threshold of resistance to irritants and an enhanced capacity for sensitization.

Household irritants not only concern substances used for the day-to-day running of the house, such as those listed in Table 11.1, but also soaps, shampoos and cosmetic or toiletry products which may be alkaline, perfumed or contain potential sensitizers. Normally well tolerated, these will penetrate a damaged epidermis and creat further irritation or induce sensitization. The possibilities here are wide and most patients do not appreciate their significance. Nickel objects, often unexpected, can be detected by a simple 'nickel testing spot test', but specialist advice and counselling is usually necessary for the patient to appreciate these hidden hazards. Certain simple precautions which can be undertaken are listed in Table 11.2 and if an occupational dermatitis persists unduly despite being off work for 2–3 weeks, one should certainly question the patient about the extent to which he or she has been following this advice.

Nickel spot test

A few drops of 1% dimethylglyoxime plus a few drops of ammonia water give a strawberry red colour. The test is extremely sensitive. Cotton buds may be used.

Soap substitutes

Emulsifying ointment BPC (also an emollient).
Unguentum Merck.
Simple Soap (Albion Co. Ltd.) } free of perfume.
Neutrogen, an original formula soap }

Gloves

PVC gloves are free of the common rubber chemicals.
Disposable polythene gloves are useful.

Climatic influences

The effects of these are underestimated. Everyone knows the effect of chapping, though 'chaps', like chilblains, have become less common with increased home warmth and better clothing. Nevertheless, an elderly worker with a dry skin who has been working in oils or solvents and who perhaps washes perfunctorily without careful rinsing and drying may suffer a chapping effect from cold winds and low humidity on his way home from work. This may be continued if his interests are outdoors. A wilting plant suffers more from a drying wind than from cold itself, and convection currents, whether cold winds or hot blow-type central heating, may desiccate and damage a skin already inflamed by work. The author believes that this is particularly important in the sequence of discoid eczema following an occupational (or a non-occupational) dermatitis. Many employees believe that their problem is due to 'dirt' or industrial contaminants and respond by increasing the frequency of their washing, with harmful results if they are getting older. The provision of after-work greasy emollients, hitherto neglected in relation to so-called 'barrier' creams, would be of great value in preventing the onset of some cases of occupational dermatitis, especially in the elderly. The continuous use of emollients might prevent the deleterious effect of these climatic factors in those who already suffer from it.

'Hidden' allergens

Unless a worker with an occupational dermatitis has been referred

Table 11.3. Some 'hidden' allergens

Formalin-releasing biocides	Soluble cutting oils Cosmetics, shampoos
Lanolin	Many cosmetics and creams, but seldom a primary occupational sensitizer
Perfumes	Complex mixtures In a great many toiletry products
Chromates, bichromate	Cement Galvanized iron Wood ash Baize table tops Primer paints etc.
Rubber chemicals	Industrial Gloves Shoe materials Rubber grips etc.

to a dermatologist with a patch testing unit, an allergic basis for his dermatitis may be overlooked. Although most engineering workers developing a dermatitis from cutting oils are probably suffering from an irritant dermatitis, it is very easy to overlook the possibility of an allergic reaction to a component of this, probably a biocide (Table 11.3). A number of these have been implicated as causes of occupational dermatitis as a result of careful patch testing to a correct dilution of the additives to the coolant, notably to formaldehyde-releasing agents or, occasionally, to mercaptobenzthiazole or chromates. The importance of determining such an allergy lies, not only in the possibility of returning the worker to his old job with an oil not containing this particular allergen, but because of continuing disability through contact with it in other forms when away from work, e.g. similar formaldehyde releasers in cosmetics and shampoos. This is a very cogent reason for early referral for full investigation of the exact cause of the eruption.

The atopic state

This has been discussed in Chapter 4. Patients with an atopic diathesis are commonly believed to be less resistant to irritants than normal subjects. They do not tolerate wool next to their skin and they more easily develop an irritant dermatitis if exposed, industrially, to potential irritants in trades such as engineering and hairdressing (Wilkinson 1975; Wilkinson & Hambly 1978). Ideally, they should be deflected early in life from such careers; but no one is anxious to take the responsibility for this. Because of the heightened reactivity of the atopic skin and the tendency for itchy areas to become easily excoriated or lichenified, an irritant occupational dermatitis in these people may pass imperceptibly into a state of chronic atopic dermatitis.

Even though there may have been no earlier history of infantile eczema, atopics may declare their diathesis later in life as a hand eczema after marriage (more housework), childbirth (nappy cleaning) or taking up a job involving contact with irritants (hairdressing, engineering, baking, cleaning, etc.). It is often difficult to know how much of the perpetuation of such an eczema is due to continued irritants at home or to the rubbing and scratching that is the inevitable accompaniment of the atopic state.

In legal terms, everyone is taken as he comes. If an atopic develops an irritant occupational dermatitis, which then continues as an 'atopic dermatitis', one has to ask oneself: would this have happened had he not been employed in this particular occupation?

Ingested allergens

There has been some interest in recent years in the possible role of allergens ingested in foods being able to cause exacerbation or provocation of eczema in those sensitive to such allergens. Attention has chiefly been directed to vesicular hand eczema in those sensitized to nickel or chromate. But the findings could presumably apply to eczema involving other sites, e.g. the eyelids. Though there is some strong experimental evidence that a dose-related reaction may indeed occur in highly sensitive subjects, the significance of this in everyday practice is disputed. Possibly the patients have to be highly sensitive and the provocative dose has usually been well in excess of the average daily intake. Most of the work has been done on nickel and it is, of course, tempting to suggest that this form of continuing exposure (though by an indirect route) might explain the frequent persistence of occupational allergic dermatitis from these metals. But it would be premature to do more than speculate at this stage. 'Low nickel' and 'low chromate' diets have been advocated but they are difficult to devise and the results are not impressive. Chelating agents are under investigation and may prove to be of help in some cases.

Medicament sensitivity

Allergic reactions to topical medicaments are responsible for most positive patch tests in Great Britain, perhaps with the exception of perfumes and nickel (in women). The frequency of such reactions is often overlooked, particularly if topical corticosteroids are being used at the same time and thus partially suppressing the reaction. In a survey of medicament sensitivity in two adjacent areas in Great Britain (Wilkinson, Hambly & Wilkinson 1980), it was shown that sensitivity to wool alcohols (lanolin) accounted for about 6% of all positive patch test reactions, and those to neomycin, parabens and ethylene diamine (a constituent of a much-used corticosteroid cream) were from 0.5 to 3%. These figures are much higher in patients being treated for leg ulcers or perianal dermatitis but they are not inconsiderable in the course of treatment of occupational dermatitis of the hands or elsewhere. Over-the-counter preparations containing 'caine' derivatives are also a common cause of an allergic sensitization. Perfumes and preservatives in proprietary and official topical preparations have been mentioned elsewhere. Especially remember preservatives in creams, e.g. ethylene diamine in one particular corticosteroid cream.

A usage test, applying a little of the preparation to the flexor surface of the forearms, twice a day for up to 3 days, may determine such a sensitivity. But standard patch test procedures are a more reliable guide. Some first-aid preparations used at the factory surgery may also be the cause of such reactions. Acriflavine still appears to be used, despite its bad record in this respect.

Cumulative damage

A first attack of occupational dermatitis will often clear up during a short period of sick leave. A second attack, if he returns to the same work, often takes longer to clear. Subsequent attacks may not clear at all, or will take very much longer to do so. The dermatitis has become 'cumulative'. This frequently happens in housewives' dermatitis.

The reason why certain individuals pass into a state of 'cumulative' dermatitis is unknown. But a successively longer period of sick leave necessary for recovery from an occupational dermatitis should be regarded as an ominous prognostic sign and every effort should be made to obtain alternative work for a patient whose recovery becomes increasingly prolonged. All other causes mentioned in this chapter should be examined; but there will remain a few workers whose dermatitis continues and eventually fails to clear, for reasons still unknown, more so in an elderly worker or one with concomitant problems of personality or anxiety.

Every effort should be made to rehabilitate him through contact with the district rehabilitation officer.

Anxiety, scratching, the 'itch–scratch' cycle

When a worker is put off work because of a rash, he naturally becomes worried and anxious on his own behalf and that of his family. Usually the eruption affects his hands and, if he is a manual worker, he feels, rightly, that he is bereft of his means to make a living. Doctors may regard hand eczema (dermatitis) as only one form of a tedious skin condition. But to a skilled manual worker (or to a housewife) it represents a major catastrophy in their lives. He often could do his job and earn his living better with an amputated leg than with a disabling hand dermatitis. To him, his hand is as important as his brain. These days there is much talk of 'quality of life' for the elderly or the infirm; but what quality of life is there for a skilled craftsman who is told that he 'must never return to that work again'?

It is no wonder that anxiety lowers the itch threshold, that he scratches and lichenifies his lesions, that secondary eczematous lesions appear as a result of the damage he does to his skin, or that infection complicates an already difficult situation.

A man of 52, working with oils and solvents, developed an irritant dermatitis of his hands. He was keen on his work but could be given no 'dry' job when his condition cleared under treatment. An attempt at returning to his old work caused a relapse. He became depressed and anxious about his future. He scratched and rubbed his lesions incessantly and developed chronic lichenified areas on his hands and forearms. He could no longer even tolerate hobbies such as gardening. He become obsessed with his condition. Four years later, in pursuance of a civil medico-legal claim, he had chronic lichenified areas of eczema for which his current treatment was quite inadequate. He was convinced that he would never be able to work again; and at this late stage of events he was probably right. But his inability to work was not a *natural* or *inevitable* consequence of his initial dermatitis. He had been left in limbo.

Self-manipulation

In a very few cases, a dermatitis will persist unduly because of deliberate manipulation by the patient. This may be on a conscious or unconscious level and, as with all artefacts, will be denied strenuously. It is not always easy to draw the line between intensive scratching in an anxious person with a low itch threshold and deliberately induced 'opening up of old wounds'. One has to sense the situation in each case. But true artefacts are more easily diagnosed by their bizarre shape or nature.

A middle-aged woman cleaner had sustained evident, straightforward irritant dermatitis of the backs of the hands but remained out of work for 14 months because, she claimed, the rash never got quite better. When examined (for medico-legal purposes) she had no evidence of eczema but a curious regular stippling of the back of one hand, compatible with the use of a stiff hairbrush. This, she claimed, came and went! And it continued to do so until the case was settled (in her favour).

Unaccountable persistence

Despite what has been said, there remain a core of patients whose eruptions persist when all the causes discussed have reasonably been excluded; often even under conditions of hospital admission. Among these, sufferers from chromate sensitivity are notorious, to the extent that these workers are just as well earning money at work with their dermatitis as they would be unemployed and still with it. A few rather rare sensitizers, e.g. some photographic chemicals, seem to produce a prolonged period of eczematous change without any possibility of further contact with the allergen. Atopic subjects have been discussed, but in the absence of any atopic or past history, an eczema may be cumulative and persistent for reasons that are quite unknown at present.

Conclusion

When an occupational dermatosis persists for more than a month after removal from the work that was allegedly responsible:

Ask

Exactly what work is he now doing?
How far away is it from his previous site of work?
What is he handling?
Is he doing any other work?
What is he doing at home (housework, gardening, decorating, other hobbies)?
Is he using soap or handling detergents or shampoos?

Is he rubbing and scratching violently?
Is he losing sleep and becoming anxious about his future?
Is he applying any over-the-counter remedies?
Is he becoming secondarily allergic to rubber gloves, lanolin, cream base preservatives, other topical medicaments?

Look

At feet (fungus).
At elbows, knees (psoriasis).
At scalp, chest, back (seborrhoeic dermatitis).
At other areas for allergic contact dermatitis (eyelids, trouser pocket area, nickel clothing clips areas, etc.).

References

Fisher A. A. (1973) *Contact Dermatitis*, 2nd edn, p. 98. Lea & Febiger, Philadelphia.

Fregert S. (1975) Occupational dermatitis in 10 year material. *Contact Dermatitis*, **1**, 96–107.

Malten K. E. (1981) Thoughts on irritant contact dermatitis. *Contact Dermatitis*, **7**, 238–247.

Wilkinson D. S. (1975) Careers advice to youths with atopic dermatitis. *Contact Dermatitis*, **1**, 11–13.

Wilkinson D. S. & Hambly E. M. (1978) Prognosis of hand eczema in hairdressing apprentices. *Contact Dermatitis*, **4**, 63.

Wilkinson J. D., Hambly E. M. & Wilkinson D. S. (1980) Comparison of patch-test results in two adjacent areas of England. II. Medicaments. *Acta Dermato-Venereologica*, **60**, 245–248.

- *Persistence of industrial dermatitis may be related to hobbies or second jobs.*
- *Bacterial or fungal infections may complicate industrial dermatitis.*
- *Physical trauma from dust, abrasives, heat and cold may intensify initial chemical damage.*
- *The skin often remains vulnerable, even though clinically normal.*
- *Premature return to the same work may be cumulatively harmful and lead to chronicity.*

Chapter 12
Chemical-induced Acne

D. M. WILLIAMSON

General aspects

The origin of the term 'acne' is obscure. The term 'acne vulgaris' was not used until 1840. This can be defined as a polymorphic skin eruption characterized clinically by blackheads (open comedones), whiteheads (closed comedones), papules, pustules, nodules, cysts and scarring occuring especially on areas of skin known to have plentiful sebaceous glands such as the face, forehead and back.

The incidence of acne vulgaris, which is predominantly a disease of adolescence which normally undergoes spontaneous resolution in adult life, has been found to vary from between 30 and 60%, with a peak incidence at 14–17 years in girls and 16–19 years in boys (Burton, Cunliffe & Stafford 1971).

Apart from acne vulgaris, there are many other types of acne, with specific features occurring at other ages and in different environmental circumstances.

Infantile acne occurs in the first few weeks of life, usually on the cheeks.

Acne conglobata is a chronic and resistant form characterized by recurrent abscess formation, irregular 'bridge type' scarring sinuses and granulomatous infiltration.

Iatrogenic acne, a chemically induced acneiform eruption, may be precipitated or aggravated by certain drugs administered orally or topically. Stimulation of testosterone secretion through gonadotrophins may induce or aggravate acne vulgaris. Anabolic steroids may do likewise. The acneiform lesions produced by corticosteroids are different in being more monomorphic and uniform in character.

Drugs containing bromide or iodide radicals and lithium may produce typical acneiform lesions. Slow inactivation of isonizid may also produce an eruption of comedones and inflammatory pustules.

Acne vulgaris appears to be more evident in patients with epilepsy and drugs given for this condition — phenobarbitone, phenytoin, hydantoin, etc. — have also been reported as provoking acne in susceptible subjects. Other drugs have occasionally been incriminated, even tetracyclines, but the evidence for this is unconfirmed.

Other causes for the development or aggravation of acne are:

Cosmetics. These have been incriminated especially in the United States. Their role is still uncertain, despite protagonists for this cause.

Friction. It is accepted that friction may induce acne lesions in predisposed subjects, e.g. coat collars and 'hand on face' in studying. Sweating and occlusion augment the effect of friction (sweat bands over the forehead, chins of violinists, etc.).

Chloracne

There are, however, a number of agents that induce an acneiform eruption by virtue of their occupational contact. These are designated by the generic term *chloracne* (Crowe 1970).

Chloracne is a disease of modern civilization, and the most important of the chemically induced acnes. It cannot be discussed fully without considering the chemistry, toxicology and the environmental aspects of the chemicals which are known to give rise to this condition. But, for the purpose of this chapter, we shall concentrate on the cutaneous aspects of the disease.

Chloracne is caused by skin contact or inhalation of certain chlorinated aromatic hydrocarbons, all of which can pass directly through intact skins, but their toxic effects are then usually less pronounced. Systemic poisoning from skin contact alone is usually accompanied by very serious chloracne.

Historical review

Chloracne was first described by Von Bettman in 1897 and later by Herxheimer in workers manufacturing hydrochloric acid. Nascent chlorine was at first thought to be responsible but it was soon accepted that the cause was related to chlorinated hydrocarbon chemicals.

In the First World War, chloracne was reported in Europe following the use of halogenated waxes containing chlorinated naphthalenes and diphenyls used in the manufacture of gasmasks.

In the 1920s and 1930s further cases of chloracne arose associated with exposure to dielectric compounds used in the electrical and radio industries. In the United States, chloracne was described in 1912 associated with the manufacture of synthetic waxes, but there was no published paper in the literature until that of Schwartz in 1936.

Waxes were used to insulate wiring loops around ships in the Second World War, to protect them from magnetic mines: chloracne occurred, in which there was marked involvement of the face, presumably due to fumes produced by heating the wax.

In the past 20 years, most cases of chloracne have been reported during the manufacture of chlorophenols, especially in the manufacture of the herbicides 2, 4, 5 trichlorophenoxyacetic acid and pentachlorphenol. It was also found that if chlorophenol was completely pure, no chloracne was produced, so that it was apparently an unwanted contaminant which was responsible for the condition. As knowledge of the contaminants increased, many of these were found to be isomeric and it was realized that some were highly toxic, and others virtually non-toxic and did not produce chloracne.

Experimental chloracne may be produced in some animals, e.g. the rhesus monkey and hairless mouse. One of the most important simple tests is the production of comedones on the inner surface of the rabbit's ear. This appears to be the most sensitive biological test surface known to date, and affords a simple and easy method of identifying an acnegenic chemical and should become a standard procedure in the evaluation of new polychlorinated aromatic hydrocarbons (Crowe 1978).

Clinical features

The eruption usually consists of a number of dense blackheads (open comedones) accompanied by the development of small pale yellow cysts of pin head size to 1 cm diameter. Many also have inflammatory papules and pustules which are often severe.

Its clinical appearance is remarkably constant, the comedones often being fine and uniform in distribution and apparently resulting from follicular hyperkeratosis. Sometimes they are so numerous that hardly a single follicle remains untouched, giving the area of affected skin a dirty grey appearance. Creamy microcysts are pathognomonic of the condition. At times skin fragility, hirsutism and hyperpigmentation also occur. The sites of election are on any exposed area of the body, especially the temporal regions, sides of neck and submandibular regions. The appearance of lesions over the malar areas of the face below and behind the pinnae are characteristic. These areas are often affected when other areas of skin are normal. Occasionally there is a preceding erythema with oedema and photosensitivity, followed by pigmentation and hyperkeratosis.

Mild cases closely resemble ordinary acne vulgaris, except for the curious concentration of blackheads and cysts around the eyes, the so-called *malar crescent*.

In all but the mildest cases, other areas of the trunk and limbs may be involved, especially where local friction occurs, e.g. over patellae, calves and around the wrists, and on the penis and scrotum. The hands and feet are usually spared.

The duration of lesions depends on the severity of the eruption, some cases still producing characteristic cropping of lesions even 15 years after the original exposure to the chloracnegen. Mild cases usually clear within months but 20% still have lesions after three years. The only severe permanent skin effect is probably associated with damage to dermal collagen (anetoderma-like scarring), usually occurring in long-standing severely affected patients.

Chloronaphthalenes

A list of chloracnegenic chemicals is shown in Table 12.1.

Chloronaphthalenes have been used as insulation materials in electrical wiring, as high pressure additives in lubricants and in wood preservatives. Many of their functions have been replaced by plastics and silicones, but in spite of this, chlorinated naphthalenes producing chloracne were described as late as 1972 in a situation where workmen were applying tetra- and pentachloronaphthalene-containing wax to insulate coils.

Crowe emphasized that chlorinated naphthalenes are very potent acnegenic agents but the degree of chlorination and the acnegenic potential are not directly related. It is thought that the most potent chloracnegens are the chloronaphthalene fumes, the

Table 12.1. Chloracnegenic chemicals

1	Chloronaphthalenes (CN)
2	Polychlorobisphenyls (PCB)
3	Polychlorinated dibenzofurans (PCF)
4	Contaminants of chlorophenols
	(a) 2, 3, 7, 8-Tetrachlorodibenzo-p-dioxin (TCDD)
	(b) Hexachlorodibenzo-p-dioxin
	(c) Tetrachlorodibenzofuran
5	Chlorobenzenes
	(a) Crude chlorobenzene
	(b) Crude benzene hexachloride
	(c) 3, 4-3, 4-Tetrachlorazoxybenzene

solids rarely causing chloracne. Chlorinated naphthalene oils and wax-like solids were manufactured in the United States under the trade name of Halowax.

An outbreak of a wasting disease affecting cattle named 'X disease' occurred in the United States and Germany during the period 1941–1954. Animals were affected with generalized follicular hyperkeratosis with dilatation and plugging of the follicles, becoming hairless and suffering a high mortality rate. The syndrome was eventually found to be due to the accidental ingestion of penta- and hexachlorinated naphthalenes. The cause appeared to be contamination of the animal foodstuff by high pressure grease containing the chloracnegen. Similar outbreaks occurred with timber preservative, again contaminated with chloracnegens, which were licked by the cattle. In Berlin in 1945 a syndrome in human subjects with gastrointestinal symptoms, oedema, erythema and choracne was found to be associated with hexachloronaphthalene contamination of fat used to fry vegetables.

Polychlorobisphenyls (PCB)

These are a series of complex compounds consisting of various polychlorinated phenyl compounds, sometimes mixed with chloronaphthalenes. The PCBs are of particular concern because their industrial use has resulted in wide dispersion and persistence of the compounds in the environment. Some PCB preparations contain the acnegenic polychlorinated dibenzofurans (BCFs) which are hepatotoxic and acnegenic.

The PCBs were used for many industrial applications, including dielectric fluids for electrical equipment, capacitators and transformers or as plastizers and heat transfer fluids, and industrial fluids for hydraulics, gas turbines and vacuum pumps.

PCBs are now only used in closed system applications and for certain specific purposes.

Several other outbreaks, involving the deaths of a large number of turkeys and chickens (Japan) have been described.

In 1968 the largest epidemic occurred in Japan, involving 1015 patients, following the ingestion of rice oil contaminated with tetrachlorobisphenyl leaking from a closed heat exchanger system in a factory manufacturing edible rice oil. There was no cutaneous contact in this outbreak which showed some unusual features in addition to a very severe chloracne affecting the face, neck and genitalia, in that a generalized follicular hyperkeratosis was seen with striking pigmentation and enlargement of the Meibomian glands. Some patients developed marked hyperkeratosis of the palms and soles and a peripheral neuropathy.

Contaminants of chlorophenols

Numerous outbreaks of chloracne have been reported during the manufacture of chlorophenols, which are primarily used as insecticides, fungicides and herbicides. In 1957, Schulz & Kimmig found a contaminant 2, 3, 7, 8-tetrachlorodibenzo-p-dioxin (TCDD) generally known as dioxin, which appeared to be formed during the synthesis of 2, 4, 5-trichlorophenol (245T). Dioxin appears to be highly toxic in humans too, e.g. 0.5 g would be lethal for 350 adults, and apart from its high toxicity it is probably the most potent chloracnegenic molecule known to date. The mechanism of action has been found to be on dividing cells where it binds with DNA. The changes may lead to possible mutation and neoplasia.

There have been recent reports of chloracne and the effects of systemic absorption of dioxin in trichlorophenol plants in France,

West Germany and Great Britain. Here, the dioxin is again produced as an unavoidable intermediate compound in the reaction because conditions of excessive pressure and temperature produce increased yields of dioxin. In these conditions the reaction becomes unstable and exothermic causing explosion of the vessel with wide scattering of the contents, producing in affected workers and persons living in the environment of the plant both severe chloracne and systemic toxicity.

One well-documented sequel of a 2, 4, 5-trichlorophenol plant explosion occurred in 1968 in a factory in Bolsover in Great Britain, resulting in 79 known cases of chloracne, many severe and presenting from a few days to several months after the explosion.

In these cases typical chloracne was seen with comedones and microcysts affecting the classical areas and also the suboccipital hair-line. Active residues may remain on clothing or equipment for many months or years.

The most recent and internationally publicized report of local and systemic dioxin toxicity occurred at Seveso in North Italy on 10 July 1976 at another 245T plant. The explosion occurred in the plant in the early morning, producing a foul-smelling cloud which drifted south contaminating the vegetation, countryside and water supply. It was thought that about 250–1000 kg of reactor fluid content escaped. The fallout contained dioxin and within days hundreds of small animals and surrounding vegetation had been destroyed. A large number of children (187) were affected initially by severe erythema on the exposed areas, thought to be due to severe primary irritation produced by sodium hydroxide and trichlorophenates in the fallout. Severe chloracne developed several weeks later showing typical features with comedones, cyst formation and marked brownish hyperkeratosis presumably indicative of severe epidermal damage. It was interesting to note that no adults were affected with chloracne although some did show evidence of polyneuropathy and hepatic enzyme changes.

As dioxin was known to be teratogenic in animals, all pregnant patients were aborted, but there was no evidence of fetal malformation. Animals in the affected zones were also slaughtered.

Dioxin is an exceedingly persistent chemical. After it had been washed off the foliage and on to the soil beneath, it tended to remain localized there.

Decontamination has consisted in removing the foliage and the top soil from the affected areas.

Chlorobenzenes

Evidence that chlorobenzenes themselves cause chloracne is sparse. Two cases have been reported after exposure to crude trichlorobenzene and benzene hydrochloride during the manufacture of DDT.

The most recent chloracnegenic agent has been identified in the report from Taylor *et al.* (1977) of an outbreak affecting 41 workers producing a herbicide VCS 438 Velsicol. Ninety percent of the workers were affected and also the children of four workers, presumably by contamination from their overalls. No porphyria or hepatoxicity was seen and the chloracnegen involved appeared to be 3, 4-3, 4-tetrachlorazoxybenzene.

An outbreak of relatively mild chloracne, affecting a number of workers, has also been described by the author, occurring in Castleford, Great Britain, in a pilot plant which had been set up to produce small quantities of Velsicol in 1972. This particular operation involved a two-stage reaction, in the second of which a toluene extraction was used. The crude toluene appeared to contain a potent acnegenic agent which was later identified as 3, 4-3, 4-tetrachloroazoxybenzene. In this episode, 22 employees developed chloracne over the malar areas, cheeks, forehead, anterior aspect of the neck and the submental and submandibular areas. A few had lesions on the buttocks and lower limbs. Reassessment of the affected patients 5 years later showed that most had cleared, but a few were still producing new lesions.

Cunliffe *et al.* (1975) investigated 12 patients from this group with chloracne and compared the data with acne vulgaris patients matched for age and sex. The ultrastructural appearance of the pilosebaceous duct keratin in both groups was identical, vacuoles which possibly contained lipid being specially prominent. Patients with chloracne showed a significant percentage increase in the surface lipids squalene, wax esters and cholesterol and these changes were associated with a significant decrease in triglycerides and fatty acids. Squalene and wax ester in the concentrations found are known to be comedogenic in animals. It was suggested that the acnegenic agent produced these changes by modifying the metabolism of the sebaceous gland. It was also found that the numbers of Micrococcaceae were similar in both forms of acne but there was significant decrease in the *P. acnes* population in the occupational group. A decrease in sebum secretion rate was also shown which is in keeping with the histological appearance of chloracne in which the sebaceous glands are often atrophic.

Toxicity

The acnegenic potential of a chemical appears to be directly related to its overall toxicity. This appears to be the case in all known chloracnegens with the possible exception of 3, 4-3, 4-tetrachloroazobenzene and possibly azobenzene.

Basic elements of the chemical structure determine the toxicity of the chloracnegens, the simplest of these being the degree of chlorination. It would appear that a chlorine content somewhere between the maximum and the minimum produces the greatest toxicity. Most important is the isomeric arrangement of the halogen atoms in their position in the molecule. Lateral symmetry in the molecule with chlorination of two adjacent carbon atoms and the presence of available hydrogen linkages all enhance toxicity. In addition to choracne disturbance of the central and peripheral nervous systems, muscle wasting, hepatic damage and hyperlipidaemia are important.

Carcinogenicity

Within the chemical industry the risk of chloracne remains, but there is no real likelihood of consumer poisoning or the development of mild chloracne from manufactured products.

From the environmental aspect, the risk of low dose long-term effects, especially cancer and damage to genetic material (mutagenicity), remains, in view of the extreme persistence of the chemicals themselves.

Experimental data on the long-term effects are confined to experimental work with the rat and mouse. PCBs produce hepatic tumours if fed in large doses throughout the animal's lifetime.

In the case of dioxin, tumours were only induced by a dosage which produced evident systemic chemical toxicity as well. With a lower non-toxic dosage no tumours were produced.

This suggests that there is a dose-related effect with regard to carcinogenicity.

Prevention

In Great Britain, 245T can be bought and used as a brushwood killer and herbicide for forest, farm and garden.

The contamination with dioxin is less than 0.1 $\mu g/g$, i.e. a guinea-pig would have to be given more than a tablespoonful of the liquid concentrate to produce any toxic effect. At the time of spraying the concentration is about 0.05 $\mu g/m^2$.

How can the risk be controlled?

Firstly, an effort must be made to publish and promulgate toxicological information widely throughout the chemical industry on an international basis.

Any new potentially related acnegenic chemical, especially if its use is intended as a pesticide or herbicide, should be tested firstly by the rabbit ear test for chloracnegenic activity, and by a comparative study made between it and a control of a known chloracnegen by the chicken enzyme test of Aryl hydrocarbon hydrolase (AHH) activity.

If a contaminant is present and responsible for the chloracnegenic potential, it may then be possible to reduce this to negligible proportions or to remove it altogether.

Only by such means of increasing people's awareness of potential acnegenic chemicals can their dangers be eliminated.

References

Burton J. L., Cunliffe W. J., & Stafford S. (1971) The prevalence of acne vulgaris in adolescence. *British Journal of Dermatology*, **85**, 119.

Crowe K. D. (1970) Chloracne. *Transactions of the St John's Hospital Dermatogical Society*, **56**, 79–99.

Crowe K. D. (1978) Chloracne — an up to date assessment. *Annals of Occupational Hygiene*, **21**, 297–198.

Cunliffe W. J., Williams M., Edwards J. C., Holland K., Roberts C., Holmes R., Williamson D. M. & Palmer W. (1975) An explanation for chloracne — an industrial hazard. *Acta Dermato-Venereologica*, **55**, 211.

Taylor J. S., Witrich R. C., Lloyd K. M. & Poland A. (1977) Chloracne from manufacture of a new herbicide. *Archives of Dermatology*, **113**, 616–619.

Chapter 13
Principles in Dermatitis Litigation

R. BURSELL

Litigation in relation to dermatitis arises in two areas:

1 Consumer protection

2 Employment

In so far as the second area is concerned there are possible claims for:

(a) Industrial injury or disablement benefit

(b) Damages

Such a damages claim may be based on breach of statutory duty or negligence or both. In each area, the medical profession may be involved prior to, or with a view to, litigation, but in either case the evidence of a doctor or consultant receives the most weight if it is given from an objective, non-partisan standpoint.

1. Consumer protection

Apart from, or in addition to, an action in negligence (see below), if personal injury is caused by a breach of contract damages may be recovered for pain and suffering if they were at the time of the contract reasonably foreseeable as liable to result from the breach.[1]

> The crucial question is whether, on the information available to the defendant when the contract was made, he should, or the reasonable man in his position would, have realised that such loss was sufficiently likely to result from the breach of contract to make it proper to hold that the loss flowed naturally from the breach or that loss of that kind should have been within his contemplation.[2]

The first question to be determined is: has there been a breach of contract? This depends upon the precise wording of each individual contract, but dermatitis cases are usually concerned with sale of goods. In any case it is for the lawyer to indicate to the doctor what the relevant question may be, e.g. whether the goods were reasonably fit for the purpose, express or implied, for which they were bought [Sale of Goods Act 1979, s.14(3)]. The question, however, is decided not by the doctor but by the judge on the evidence given by the doctor. In the main, that evidence will be concerned with two problems:

1 how was the dermatitis caused (causation)?

2 was it foreseeable that it would be caused by the breach of contract (forseeability)?

In so far as causation is concerned, it may be possible to point to the facts as raising an evidential presumption in favour of the consumer. For example, in *Mayne* v. *Silvermere Cleaners Ltd*[3] it was held that, when dermatitis was contracted after wearing a professionally cleaned suit, it was for the cleaners to show that they were not to blame.

As to foreseeability, in *Grant* v. *Australian Knitting Mills Ltd*[4] where it was not contemplated by the parties that the underpants would be washed before use, the manufacturers were held liable for damages in relation to dermatitis caused by a chemical irritant in the underwear. However, in *Griffiths* v. *Peter Conway Ltd*[5] the plaintiff, who had had a coat especially made for her, failed to recover damages for dermatitis caused by the Harris Tweed, as the cloth would not have affected the skin of a normal person. The result would have been different if she had made known to the manufacturer the fact that she had abnormally sensitive skin.[6]

2. Employment

A. Industrial injury or disablement benefit

By reason of the Social Security Act 1975, s.56 (1), an employed earner is entitled to injury benefit in respect of any day during the injury benefit period on which, as a result of the relevant injury, he or she is incapable of work. However,

> non-infective dermatitis of external origin (including chrome ulceration of the skin but excluding dermatitis due to ionising particles or electro-magnetic radiations other than radiant heat)

is a disease prescribed by the Secretary of State in relation to

> any occupation involving exposure to dust, liquid or vapour or any other external agent capable of irritating the skin (including friction or heat but excluding ionising particles or electro-magnetic radiations other than radiant heat).[7]

If an employed earner suffers from such a dermatitis he may claim injury benefit just as if he had suffered an accident at work: Social Securities Act 1975, s.77(1). He must therefore show

1 that he suffers from such a non-infective dermatitis;
2 that his occupation involves the necessary exposure;
3 that the dermatitis developed as a result of his occupation.

1. *Non-infective dermatitis.* This is primarily a medical question and an appeal lies from the medical board to a medical appeal tribunal. However, provided he otherwise fulfils the necessary criteria, an employee is treated as though he is suffering from the prescribed dermatitis if he has a condition resulting from it: Social Security (Industrial Injuries) (Prescribed Diseases) Regulations 1975, reg.3. Moreover, any recrudescence within the injury benefit period gives no further entitlement unless medical evidence shows it to be a fresh attack; it may nevertheless be grounds for a review of the original assessment.

2. *Necessary exposure.* The claimant must be actually working in the relevant occupation rather than being incidentally involved with it. It is sufficient if the involvement is an accepted, but not necessarily major, part of his work — an 'accepted concomitant' rather than a 'voluntary task'.[8] Nonetheless the time spent in the relevant occupation is less important than its regularity.

3. *Dermatitis as a result of occupation.* The claimant must prove that the dermatitis developed as a result of his occupation. Causation is therefore of prime importance as, unlike most prescribed diseases, there is no presumption of such causation to assist him.[9]

If as a result of the prescribed dermatitis an employed earner suffers any loss of physical or mental faculty of not less than 1%, disablement benefit may be claimed: Social Security Act 1975, s.57(1). Physical faculty includes disfigurement. Industrial injury and disablement benefits cannot be received at the same time and, once disablement benefit has been awarded, injury benefit can no longer be claimed.

B. Damages[10]

Whereas a claim for benefits is concerned with a purely causative connection between the dermatitis and the relevant employment, a claimant for damages must in addition show that his dermatitis arose from a breach of statutory duty owed to him or of a general duty to take care (negligence).

Breach of statutory duty

At first sight the employer's duty under section 1[11] of the Factories Act 1961[12] adds nothing to the general duty to take care in a normal factory situation:

> Every factory shall be kept in a clean state ...

Nevertheless, the distinction may be important in that the plaintiff, having proved the breach, need only prove that on a balance of probabilities the breach caused or materially contributed to his injury.[13] The same is also true of section 29 which provides that

> ... every place at which any person has at any time to work ... shall, so far as is reasonably practicable, be made and kept safe for any person working there.

It is for the employer to prove that he has taken all reasonably practical steps,[14] and

> it cannot be reasonable to do ... anything more than that which it appears necessary and sufficient to do according to the best assessment of what is necessary and sufficient that can be made at the relevant time.[15]

Reliance may also be placed[16] on section 4,

> Effective and suitable provision shall be made for securing and maintaining by circulation of fresh air in each workroom the adequate ventilation of the room, and for rendering harmless, so far as practicable[17] all such fumes, dust and other impurities generated in the course of any process or work carried on in the factory as may be injurious to health

or section 63(1),[18]

> In every factory in which, in connection with any process carried on, there is given off any dust or fume or other impurity of such a character and to such extent as to be likely to be injurious or offensive to the persons employed, or any substantial quantity of dust of any kind, all practicable measures shall be taken to protect the persons employed against inhalation of the dust or fume or other impurity and to prevent its accumulating in any workroom ...

Nevertheless, most frequently, reliance is placed on section 58,[19]

> There shall be provided and maintained for the use of employed persons adequate and suitable facilities for washing which shall include a supply of clean running hot and cold or warm water and, in addition, soap and clean towels or other suitable means of cleaning or drying; and the facilities shall be conveniently accessible and shall be kept in a clean and orderly condition.

In practice this section often does little more than help to delimit the employer's duties at common law. For example, in *Wishart* v. *Bradley & Craven Ltd*[20] a workman contracted dermatitis from chemically impregnated sand. The employers were held not to be in breach of section 58 as they had provided adequate washing facilities at a distance of 70 yards, whereas at the plaintiff's actual place of work there was merely a cold water tap. The Court of Appeal held that at the relevant time dermatitis was not reasonably foreseeable and the employers could not be negligent in doing more than the statute required.

Duty to take care

Although it is for a plaintiff to prove his case on a balance of probabilities he may be able to rely upon an evidential presumption to assist him in proving causation.

> When a man who has not previously suffered from a disease contracts that disease after being subjected to conditions likely to cause it, and when he shows that it starts in a way typical of disease caused by such conditions, he establishes a prima facie presumption that his disease was caused by those conditions.[21]

Nevertheless such an evidential burden may at any time be displaced.[22] Moreover, the gravamen is whether the conditions were 'likely to cause' the dermatitis. If other workmen on the same job and in similar circumstances have not contracted dermatitis the presumption may be displaced.

The employer is under a duty towards his employee to take 'reasonable care in all the circumstances'[23] or, in other words,

> to provide proper appliances, and to maintain them in a proper condition, and so to carry on his operations as not to subject those employed by him to unnecessary risk.[24]

The general principle is that[25]

> a person must be regarded as negligent if he does not take steps to eliminate a risk which he knows or ought to know is a real risk and not a mere possibility which would never influence the mind of a reasonable man.

It follows that the taking of proper precautions — proper, that is, for a person with normal skin — in relation to a known sensitizer or known primary irritant eliminates liability whereas failure to take them creates liability. If an employee develops dermatitis in spite of such precautions, he cannot recover damages. Similarly he cannot recover if he contracts dermatitis from a substance not known to be a sensitizer or primary irritant; in such cases there is no foreseeable risk against which to take precautions. On the other hand, if an employer wishes to introduce a new substance, to escape liability he must make reasonable enquiries before introducing it. If, however, the employer has exposed an employee to a substance or circumstances which may act as a primary irritant, such as mild irritants, heat friction or work trauma, to succeed the employee must show that the degree and nature of contact was such that the employer should have foreseen the risk to the skin of a normal person in the absence of precautions and should have taken those precautions.[26] It remains, however, to consider the cases of an employee's own particular sensitivity. In *Clayton* v. *Caledonia Stevedoring Co.*[27] an employer was held not to be liable to an employee who contracted dermatitis from handling ammonium chloride because the latter, unknown to the employer, had a hypersensitive skin. An employee is under a duty to inform his employer if he knows he is abnormally susceptible;[28] similarly an employer must take extra precautions in relation to an employee whom he knows or ought to know has a particular sensitivity.[29] As Sir Wilfrid Green MR said in *Griffiths* v. *Peter Conway Ltd*,[30]

> ... I am not ... referring to any variations which take place and exist within the class of normal people. No two normal people are precisely alike, and, in the matter of sensitiveness of skin, among people who would be described as normal their sensitiveness must vary in degree. This does not mean that there is a line which it is the function of the court, or of a medical witness, to draw with precision, so as to define all cases where normality ceases and abnormality begins. The impossibility of drawing such a line by reference to some scientific formula or something of that kind does not mean that, for the present purpose, the difference between normality and abnormality is a thing that must be disregarded or cannot be ascertained.

Nevertheless, the reasonable employer should err on the side of safety as he must cater for employees who are 'normal in their sensitivity, or, at any rate, not altogether exceptional'.[31]

It does not follow, however, that an employee with a particular susceptibility cannot be employed or continue to be employed. An employer in a direct irritant case may in response to medical advice keep an employee at a job for a reasonable period after the dermatitis has been diagnosed in an attempt to harden his skin to that job. Moreover,[32]

> It cannot be said that an employer is bound to dismiss an employee rather than allow her to run a small risk. The employee is free to decide for herself what risks she will run . . . If the employer were to conceal the risk or fail to give the employee information which he had and which might help to evaluate it properly, there might perhaps be a liability; or I suppose there might be a case in which an employer impliedly warranted that job was safe for a particular employee.

Evidence

It has already been emphasized that any medical evidence should be as impartial as possible. Clearly, too, care must be taken to retail in any medical reports a detailed and accurate history and description of the dermatitis and especially its first manifestations. Such a history is often critical and for this reason actual quotations from the patient himself may be of great importance.

It should be borne in mind that different considerations apply in industrial injury or disablement cases on the one hand and actions for damages on the other. It is therefore essential that a medical expert should be asked to reconsider such cases and that he should report again if a civil claim is to be made. Quite apart from the difference in approach this will give the expert an opportunity to consider the up-to-date position and alter, or entirely change, his view if necessary. It is also essential that any groundwork, such as an investigation into the chemical properties of a cutting oil or any additive, should be carried out prior to trial.

Finally it should be borne in mind that each individual case depends upon the evidence given in it. Thus in *Clifford* v. *Charles H. Challen & Son Ltd*[33] the employer was found liable in negligence for not providing a barrier cream, having displayed a notice recommending its use, whereas in *Brown* v. *Rolls Royce Ltd*[34] the employers, who had accepted the advice of their medical officer which did not include the use of barrier cream, were held not to be negligent although it was proved that a type of barrier cream was commonly supplied by employers to men doing such work. It is therefore important that any medical report should deal with all aspects of the individual case (as well as common practice, if relevant) together with the expert's medical opinion on each aspect, such as the effectiveness of barrier creams or the effect of bacteria in cutting oils. If such evidence is not given subsequently at court, the fault will then lie with the lawyers and not with the expert concerned.

Notes

1 *Victoria Laundry (Windsor) Ltd* v. *Newman Industries Ltd* [1949] 2 KB 528 at 539. It is unnecessary that the parties themselves should foresee the breach: *Christopher Hill Ltd* v. *Ashington Piggeries Ltd* [1969] 3 All ER 1496 at 1523. The colloquialism 'on the cards' should not be used: *Koufos* v. *C. Czarnikow Ltd* [1969] 1 AC 350 at 390, 399, 415 & 425.
2 *Koufos* v. *C. Czarnikow Ltd* [1969] 1 AC 350 at 385.
3 [1939] 1 All ER 693.
4 [1936] AC 85.
5 [1939] 1 All ER 685.
6 *Ingham* v. *Emes* [1955] 2 QB 366, where a customer who knew she was allergic to a particular hair dye, failed to warn the hairdresser.
7 Social Security (Industrial Injuries) (Prescribed Diseases) Regulations 1975 (SI No. 1537) schedule 1, as amended.
8 National Insurance Commissioner's Decisions, R(1) 8/57; see, generally, *Social Welfare Law*, ed. Pollard, Vol. 1, Part D, Chap. 5.
9 Social Security (Industrial Injuries) (Prescribed Diseases) Regulations 1975, reg. 4, as amended.
10 See the admirable article by Peter Fallon, QC, LLB (now His Honour Judge Fallon) in *Proceedings of the Royal Society of Medicine*, **65**, 33.
11 Breach of the section gives rise to a civil claim: *Carroll* v. *North British Locomotive Co.* [1957] SLT (Sh.Ct.) 2.
12 Breach of the Health and Safety at Work Act 1974 incurs no civil liability: s.47.
13 *Bonnington Castings Ltd* v. *Wardlaw* [1956] AC 613; *McGhee* v. *National Coal Board* [1973] 1 WLR 1. It is material unless it is 'so negligible that the maxim '*de minimis*' is applicable': *Nicholson* v. *Atlas Steel Co. Ltd* [1957] 1 All ER 776 at 781.
14 *Gibson* v. *British Insulated Callender's Construction Co. Ltd* 1973 SLT 2: *Bowes* v. *Sedgefield District Council* [1981] ICR 234.
15 *Marshall* v. *Gotham* [1954] AC 360 at 370 (citing [1953] 1 QB 167 at 179) 'There may well be precautions which it is 'practicable' but not 'reasonably practicable' to take': op. cit. at 373. 'Practicable' means capable of being carried out in action or 'feasible': *Lee* v. *Nursery Furnishings Ltd* [1945] 1 All ER 387 at 389.
16 See *Graham* v. *Co-operative Wholesale Soc. Ltd* [1957] 1 All ER 654.
17 See note 15.
18 See *Graham* v. *Co-operative Wholesale Soc. Ltd* [1957] 1 All ER 654.
19 The section gives rise to a civil claim: *Reid* v. *Westfield Paper Co. Ltd* [1957] SC 218. But see *Clifford* v. *Charles H. Challen & Son Ltd* [1951] 1 KB 496.
20 [1963] 107 SJ 554.
21 *Gardiner* v. *Motherwell Machinery and Scrap Co. Ltd* [1961] 3 All ER 831 at 832.

22 See *Brown* v. *Rolls-Royce Ltd* [1960] 1 All ER 577.
23 *Cavanagh* v. *Ulster Weaving Co. Ltd* [1960] AC 145 at 167.
24 *Smith* v. *Charles Baker & Sons* [1891] AC 325 at 362.
25 *Wagon Mound (No. 2)* [1967] 1 AC 617 at 642 per Lord Reid.
26 See the article by His Honour Judge Fallon cited in note 10.
27 (1948) 81 L1. L. Rep. 332.
28 *Cork* v. *Kirby Maclean* [1952] 2 All ER 402.
29 *Paris* v. *Stepney Borough Council* [1951] AC 367.
30 [1939] 1 All ER 685 at 691–692.
31 *Board* v. *Thomas Hedley & Co. Ltd* [1951] 2 All ER 431 at 432.
32 *Withers* v. *Perry Chain Co. Ltd* [1961] 3 All ER 676 at 680; *Kossinski* v. *Chrysler United Kingdom Ltd* (1974) 15 KIR 225.
33 [1951] 1 KB 495.
34 [1960] 1 All ER 577.

Appendixes

1. Further reading list

Adams R. M. (1969) *Occupational Contact Dermatitis*. J. P. Lippincott, Philadelphia. A standard work, straightforward and easily understood text.

Cronin E. (1980) *Contact Dermatitis*. Churchill Livingstone, Edinburgh. A very comprehensive account of allergens recognized to this date, and their sources, frequency of sensitivity and clinical presentation.

Fisher A. A. (1973) *Contact Dermatitis*, 2nd edn. Lea & Febiger, Philadelphia. For many years a standard source of reference on all aspects of contact hypersensitivity.

Foussereau J., Benezra C. & Maibach H. I. (1982) *Occupational Contact Dermatitis: Clinical and Chemical Aspects*. Munksgaard, Copenhagen. A useful recently updated addition to the literature.

Fregert S. (1981) *Manual of Contact Dermatitis*. Munksgaard, Copenhagen. A short text with many useful tips.

Hjorth N. & Fregert S. (1985) Contact dermatitis. In *Textbook of Dermatology*, 4th edn (eds A. Rook, D. S. Wilkinson and F. J. G. Ebling). Blackwell Scientific Publications, Oxford.
A well-referenced monograph in itself, in a widely accepted two-volume general textbook of dermatology.

Maibach H. I. & Gellin G. A. (1982) *Occupational and Industrial Dermatology*. Year Book Medical Publishers Inc., Chicago.
A compact and easily assimilated textbook on the subject.

Malten K. E., Nater J. P. & van Ketel W. G. (1976) *Patch Test Guidelines*. Dekker & Van de Vegt, Nijmegen.
A small systematic and invaluable guide.

Nater J. P., de Groot A. C. & Liem D. H. (1983) *Unwanted Effects of Cosmetics and Drugs used in Dermatology*. Excerpta Medica, Amsterdam.
Many sections of interest in the industrial field.

All large industrial medical centres should consider subscribing to

Contact Dermatitis, the journal of environmental and occupational dermatitis (ed. C. D. Calnan)
Issued bi-monthly, Munksgaard, Copenhagen.

2. Common sources of occupational dermatitis

Males

Order of importance	Occupation	Common allergens	Common irritants
1	Metal industry	Rubber, chromium, plastics	Solvents, hand cleansing agents, oils
2	Cement casting	Chromium, cobalt, rubber gloves	Cement, oils
3	Building industry	Chromium, cobalt, rubber gloves, epoxy resin, leather (chromium) gloves	Cement, wood preservatives
4	Plastics industry	Resins, hardeners	Plastics, solvents, fibre glass
5	Woodwork	Woods, plastics	Plastics
6	Rubber industry	Rubber chemicals	Solvents, hand cleansing agents
7	Food industry	Rubber gloves, vegetables	Cleaning agents, vegetables, fish, meat, fruit
8	Car repair industry	Rubber, chromium, nickel	Oils, solvents, hand cleansing agents
9	Agriculture	Plants, rubber gloves, leather (chromium) gloves, medicaments for animals, feed additives	Oils, solvents, fertilizers, cleansing agents
10	Painting	Chromium, turpentine, glue, epoxy resin	Solvents, hand cleansing agents, paints, glues

Females

Order of importance	Occupation	Common allergens	Common irritants
1	Cleaning	Rubber gloves, nickel	Cleaning agents
2	Hospital	Rubber gloves, nickel, medicaments, antiseptics	Cleaning agents
3	Hairdressing	Nickel, hair dyes, rubber gloves, perfumes	Shampoos, permanent wave solutions, oxidizing agents, bleaching agents
4	Food industry	Rubber gloves, vegetables	Cleaning agents, vegetables, fish, meat, fruit
5	Hotel/ restaurant	Nickel, vegetables	Cleaning agents, food
6	Rubber industry	Rubber chemicals	Solvents, hand cleansing agents
7	Plastics industry	Resins, hardeners	Plastics, solvents, fibre glass
8	Textile industry	Textile dyes, nickel, formaldehyde	Solvents, bleaching agents
9	Laboratory	Chemicals	Solvents, alkalis, acids
10	Nursery/ florists	Plants, pesticides	Fertilizers

3. European Standard 'battery'

Most large centres belonging to the European Contact Dermatitis Research Group (ECDRG) use very similar lists of standard contact allergens as a 'battery' for patch testing. That recommended currently by the ECDRG is given below. To this standard battery, additional patch tests are usually added according to the patient's occupational and other exposures.

ES no.	Reagent	Concentration
1	Potassium dichromate	0.5%
2	p-Phenylene diamine (PPD)	0.5%
3	Thiuram mix (4 at 0.25%)	1%
4	Neomycin sulphate	20%
5	Cobalt chloride	1%
6	Benzocaine	5%
7	Nickel sulphate	5%
8	Quinoline mix	6%
9	Colophony	60%
10	Parabens (5 at 3%)	15%
11	PPD mix (Black rubber mix)	0.6%
12	Wool alcohols	30%
13	Mercapto mix (4 at 0.5%)	2%
14	Epoxy resin	1%
15	Balsam of Peru	25%
16	Paratertiary butylphenol formaldehyde resin	1%
17	Carba mix (3 at 1%)	3%
18	Formaldehyde (in water)	1%
19	Fragrance mix (8 at 1%)	8%
20	Ethylene diamine dihydrochloride	1%
21	Cis-1-(3-chloroally)-3,5,7-triaza-1-aziona-adamantane chloride (Quaternium 15)	1%
22	Primin	0.01%

Index